How To Be
Healthier, Wealthier, Happy and Wise

What You Need To Know To Be Healthy

Kathleen Babbitt, D.Sc.

toExcel
San Jose New York Lincoln Shanghai

How to Be Healthier, Wealthier, Happy and Wise
What You Need To Know To Be Healthy

This edition published by toExcel Press,
an imprint of iUniverse.com, Inc.

For information address:
iUniverse.com, Inc.
620 North 48th Street
Suite 201
Lincoln, NE 68504-3467
www.iuniverse.com

ISBN: 0-595-00142-4

This book is dedicated to everyone I have known who has suffered unnecessarily -- emotionally, mentally, physically, spiritually.

INTRODUCTION

This book tells you about things which none of us, anywhere, can avoid. The poisoning of the Earth, the air, the water, and ourselves, was not inevitable, is not inevitable even at this late date, if we do something -- many things -- to change it. My book was written to capsulize these problems as they relate to individuals everywhere, and to summarize solutions on an individual level to the health problems they create.

At the center of this approach is holistic medicine and lifestyles. Holistic means to integrate all facets of life, all parts of living healthfully, and acknowledging the interrelatedness of all life. The holistic medical approach finds and corrects the underlying reasons instead of suppressing the symptoms with drugs or surgical removal.

One imbalance leads to another, and another, indefinitely. Doctors know, as an example, that hysterectomies and removal of ovaries cause an increase in heart disease and breast cancer. Doctors know that about 90% of hysterectomies are unnecessary. Therefore, doctors are indirectly and directly responsible for the death and suffering and diminishing of the quality of life of millions of women. For this liability of untold suffering or despair they are paid royally. This, in turn, creates arrogance and greed and disrespect for women. All of this makes the Hippocratic Oath a joke.

In the U.S. an average of 200 people die every day because of doctor mistakes. Malpractice suits are not an answer. It is very difficult to prove malpractice. Anyway, that is after-the-fact, after the damage has been done. The perpetuation of the Western medical system is of course dependent on public use and acceptance.

Pablo Picasso said, "When you come right down to it, all you have is yourself. The rest is nothing." Although I think this is rather myopic, there are elements of truth and reality in it. However, begin to heal yourself and you begin to heal the world. The interrelatedness of all living things begins with yourself.

CBS News reported that more than half of all Americans use health care outside the medical norm. This book supplements this growing demand for natural healing. It's about health problems and their causes, and solutions that are natural, safe, and easy. Ways to help the body heal itself.

Millions of Americans want to be healthier. Many people want natural solutions to their health problems. In this book you will discover the hidden reasons people are not healthy and you will learn proven natural solutions to get healthy and stay healthy. Domination over Nature is not an answer.

By a child's first birthday the cancer risk from pesticides exceeds the EPA's lifetime levels of acceptable risk. The relationship of our health to the environment we live in needs to be known by everyone. Natural and holistic therapies provide some solutions to the health problems created by an unhealthy environment.

Drugs/chemicals attempt to overpower, control, and eliminate. Healing with natural and holistic therapies is synergistic, life enhancing, and harmonious with life. At this time in history we have more potential choices than ever before for methods of health care.

An ailing America needs catalysts for this very important, simple knowledge. Individually and together we can do what is right and good.

Buddhists believe suffering exists to teach compassion, and the middle way, compassion, is the best spiritual and mental attitude because it's centered. Self-poisons are doubt, shame, fear, depression, hostility, anger, grief, anxiety, and greed. To be happier replace these harmful emotions with those that have the power to heal: appreciation, acceptance, love, hope, humor, enthusiasm, tolerance, and patience. Also, look at problems as opportunities, and don't be judgemental. But causes of many mental and emotional problems can be toxicity, allergies, nutritional imbalances and deficiencies, and no amount of positive thinking or counseling or compassion can correct that.

I wrote this book to help every individual who reads it to begin to help himself or herself to be completely healthy. And then help their world around them be completely healthy -- wherever, whatever, whoever, that might be.

Together we can do it. As Margaret Mead, anthropologist, said: "Thoughtful, committed citizens can change the world. Indeed, it's the only thing that ever has. "

Good Luck!

CHAPTER I
AN OVERVIEW

For about half a century there have been knowledgeable people able to lead others to a sickness free life. This same simple knowledge has been able to cure cancer, asthma, allergies, arthritis, diabetes (not dependent on insulin), digestion problems, gallbladder and liver problems, high blood pressure, heart disease, overweight, skin problems (acne, psoriasis etc.), rheumatism, headaches, insomnia, hyperactive behavior, other so-called behavior problems, etc. It is preferable, of course, and possible, to avoid these health problems, but often they can be alleviated after onset through natural healing.

Natural healing is non-toxic, inexpensive, has a high cure rate, and can be understood by anyone. Approximately 90% of all sicknesses can be helped. Eliminate deficiencies and excesses that allowed sickness to develop, that caused disease, and then rebuild through diet, and possibly vitamins, minerals, enzymes, amino acids, essential fatty acids, and other appropriate supplementation.

Millions of people diagnosed as "incurable" needlessly die each year. They do not, or did not, use principles of natural healing and regeneration.

Dr.Max Gerson provided proof to a subcommittee of the United States Senate in July of 1946 that a high micronutrient diet with salt and water management, and a program of detoxification, cured many diverse conditions, including those previously mentioned. Dr.Albert Schweitzer said, "I see in Dr.Max Gerson one of the most eminent geniuses in medical history." The

Gerson Institute is in California, but the hospital for therapy and treatment is in Tijuana, Mexico.

Why haven't these methods of natural healing and regeneration been made common knowledge? This book explores the issues behind this disturbing phenomenon, and presents some answers. Also, it is a comprehensive guide to better health.

*****

Dr. A.J. Shadman, M.D., said, "After 40 years observation of the inefficiencies and awful blunders of physicians I do not believe I exaggerate when I say that orthodox medicine is killing more people yearly than war and disease combined."

The causes of disease are excesses. Getting well and staying well become so much simpler when you understand this. When you discontinue and remove all causes of disease you'll enjoy sickness-free health. The best defense is to eliminate disease causing influences. But this is easier said than done.

Something as simple and common as digestive problems has an easy remedy -- eat foods together that are compatible in digestive chemistry. Do not mix types of food, groups of food. But it is human nature to be unwilling to change dietary habits and patterns. (Even if it would mean avoidance of unpleasant digestive problems!) Unfortunately, the food you like best may be the worst for you. You may be addicted to harmful food, like alcohol or cigarette addiction.

One of the disadvantages of living in a modern society becomes apparent when we try to make life easier by indulging in convenience foods, which are usually full of chemicals, and therefore harmful for us. Along the same approach to life are people's reactions to medical problems, health problems. People want a quick (convenient) recovery, with no major changes in their lifestyle or diet. This strong aversion to dietary change must be overcome to begin a cure, to become truly and enduringly healthy, which is everyone's birthright.

* * * * *

Every person in the U.S. deserves to have access to health promotion and prevention of disease. Insurance and Medicare/Medicaid do not pay for preventive care services. Doctors do not make nearly as much money preventing as they do caring for after the problem has occurred. What would happen to hospitals and their highly paid staff if our medical system was prevention oriented, instead of illness oriented? The promotion of healthier lifestyles would reduce the need for many high-cost medical procedures. Americans spent nearly a trillion dollars on health care in 1995. Yes, nearly a trillion dollars. In the U.S. more is spent on health care per person than *any* other country. Yet, our infant mortality rate is 22nd among 24 developed countries. Repeated studies have revealed many medical procedures are being performed unnecessarily and increasingly. In 1990, the U.S. spent more than $2500 per person for health care, *double* the amount of other industrialized countries that provide health care coverage to *all* of their citizens. Millions of Americans have *no* health coverage. More than 40 million, to be exact. American corporations spend an average of $3452 a year per employee for health care. Japanese corporations pay roughly $700 per employee. This affects our ability to compete in the world market.

Ever increasing health care costs take away from government funds available for other social needs. Less money is available for jobs, education, and public works.

Are you satisfied with a health care system like this? If not, write Congressmen, Senators, etc. Don't pay for unnecessary medical procedures. Take responsibility for your health. Complain about hugely inflated costs. Don't be a victim of an unfair, cost-inflated, too often ineffective and mistake ridden system.

As an example, 90% of hysterectomies, with or without removal of ovaries, are unnecessary. They have been referred to as "cash cows" for the medical establishment. In the U.S. about 750,000 women a year suffer unnecessarily from this very painful operation. That's three-quarters of a million women. In ten years that's 7.5 million women, ad infinitum. Repeatedly, statistics have shown that normal health is an impossibility for many women for an indefinite period of time (maybe never) after this destructive surgery. Ten percent of women who have it need it to save their lives, the other 90% should be given alternative approaches. (Even acupuncture is an alternative.) A high percentage of women have complications during and after, even years after, the surgery. (About 600 women die yearly.) Quality of life is usually diminished. Would male doctors castrate three-quarters of a million men a year if the danger of cancer for them was .5%? Of course not. Yet, that is the risk of ovarian cancer -- one-half of 1%, for which doctors routinely remove ovaries during a hysterectomy.

Physiological balance is impossible for most women after this surgery. The complete interplay of all hormones supplied by the ovaries and uterus cannot be duplicated by synthetic estrogen, progesterone, or horse urine

10

(Premarin). A naturally post-menopausal woman continues to produce small amounts of estrogen, androgen, and progesterone from the uterus and ovaries. (For more information read *The Hysterectomy Hoax* and *No More Hysterectomies.*) Unnecessary hysterectomies are added to heart bypass surgery and chemotherapy as a huge source of unnecessary pain and misery for patients, and as a gigantic source of money for the medical establishment. We are not beneficiaries, we are victims.

In holistic medicine the whole patient is regarded. The interrelationship of all parts of the whole person -- mind, body, spirit -- are all taken into account. Conventional medicine often fails, while guidance, counseling, and alternative medicine often succeed. As Plato said, "Do not separate the soul, or spirit, from the body in treatment."

Old practices, treatments, and remedies dormant for a long time are being rediscovered. European nature cures called "Kniepp cures" involve hydration therapy, sunshine, exercise and diet that is wholesome and uncooked. In the Philippines, healing is sometimes accomplished by putting the left hand behind the head, and the right hand on the forehead, or pain source, by revered healers held in high esteem by the local population. This sounds bizarre and unbelievable, but often works. Perhaps it's a case of mind over matter, absolute belief in the healer's abilities, or mind control. Without a doubt, a positive attitude is important in the healing process. Everyone can replace negative thoughts with positive thoughts and benefit.

During the healing process the body throws off its toxic accumulation by an acute crisis, which manifests as a disease or sickness. Therefore, to be sick is a step towards being well again, as the body tries to restore balance.

11

During this process even an aspirin can be harmful, as the aspirin lessens the fever -- a natural part of healing, i.e. ridding the body of toxic accumulation by increasing white cells and antibodies.

One imbalance leads to another. As an example, overweight leads to other health problems. Most people over the age of about 35 digest and utilize only about 30% to 50% of anything they ingest. This explains why vitamins and supplements don't do as much good after that age, and why middle age is synonymous with fat accumulation and fatigue. This explains why we need to eat more and more food to satisfy our hunger, and why that undigested food turns to fat. Our overall health can be measured by our digestive capabilities.

Take time to be well, instead of letting sickness take time away from you. Get rid of accumulated wastes and toxins before health can be restored. Incomplete digestion, bowel toxemia, impaired liver function, refined and processed food, chemicals in our food, air, and water, are causes of many health problems. For optimum health get rid of the causes.

"The body heals itself when the causes for its problems are eliminated." said Dr. Shelton, author of books and articles on the subject of fasting and natural health.

*****

CHAPTER II
THE POISONING OF AMERICA

Cosmic energy is a prime force for life and its functions. Everything is energy; life is energy. Disease and sickness are imbalances or deviations from the norm. With chronic, or incurable, diseases and sicknesses it is important to immediately start the process of restoration, not destruction, to restore and increase energy within the body to facilitate health. Herbs have life forces concentrated in them, energy forces. Drugs, pharmaceuticals, do not. Anti-biotics means "anti-life." (They kill beneficial bacteria along with harmful bacteria.)

Organically grown fruits and vegetables have life forces-- energy forces -- within them, if they are fresh and raw. The liver produces life and energy if it is healthy. If it isn't, health problems are inevitable, as it struggles with adversity that is unnecessary.

The leading principle of the natural approach to health is a return to Hippocrates' precept "Above all, do not damage."

People must practice a balanced way of life to restore to normal conditions. Unfortunately, "normal" is becoming "abnormal" more and more frequently. Conversely, facets and standards of health which were once considered "abnormal" are now "normal," or common. It is only when the body recovers its general balance that painful problems disappear.

Chemically contaminated food and air and water destroy energy and health. Even cooked food destroys health and energy because heat above 118° F kills living organisms.

13

Dr. Butterworth, of the University of Alabama, said, "There's a need to find the most economical way to treat and prevent chronic disease." There is one that has been known for decades -- the holistic or naturalist way, as chronicled in many books and reports.

However, medical and pharmaceutical establishments have vested interests in condemning it, despite many hundreds of case histories proving its success. Also do the milk and dairy food industries, and the meat industries. And, of course, the processed food industries. You must take responsibility for your own health, and of those you love, and persevere in spite of huge industries, i.e. money interests, working against true health.

The worst culprit of all, causing disease and sickness perpetuation and creation, is the vast chemical industry. It's like a giant monster, spreading death and destruction slowly, insipidly, everywhere, or suddenly anywhere. Chemicals have worldwide ramifications, and often do not dissipate completely for many years -- sometimes thousands of years.

As an example, although atom bombs and nuclear bombs were detonated repeatedly in <u>Nevada</u>, hundreds of them since the 1940's, people living in St.George,<u>Utah</u> reported mushroom clouds of nuclear or atomic waste over their town. White particles would fall onto their yards and houses from these clouds, and their children would play in it like it was snow. The United States Government had repeatedly assured them it was harmless. However, the Government and Army changed the positioning and pattern of bombing in Nevada so the deadly chemical clouds and chemical "snow" falls stopped in St.George, Utah. As the years passed, people were dying from cancers at an alarming rate, much higher than the

14

national average.   Children were dying of cancer and leukemia. Newborn children had leukemia.

Some of the chemicals in atomic and nuclear bombs have a destructive "life" of a thousand or more years. Other chemical components of nuclear and atomic bomb wastes only have a "life" of hundreds of years.   Still, others have less than a hundred.

* * * * *

Pesticides upset normal nutritional balances in fruit and vegetables.   Disease organisms and bacteria spread rapidly through the weakened fruit, necessitating more and different pesticides. This is similar to antibiotics which eventually don't work on the problems they were designed to solve. This endless pesticide cycle produces nutritionally unfit vegetables or fruit, covered with poison.   Pesticides and antibiotics found in our food supply, alone, can be enough to upset the bacteria balance in the digestive tract, hampering nutrient absorption.

In *How to Prevent Pesticide Pollution* Jeffery Dearborn says, "We look to science for solutions, yet if science could save us, it would be cleaning up the environment, and the results would be less cancers, not more."

Using pesticides, fertilizers, and fumigants to excess creates a system that is out of balance. In this depleted soil environment plants don't produce safe, nutritious food. When vegetables and fruit are sick, then so are we. What we get from our crops are less nutrition and more cancer.

Are chemical companies and farmers going to continue to poison the Earth for profits, for greed? We all know they will. So we are pawns in this monstrous game.

15

We all know that there are safe, simple methods the entire food industry can use but does not, because these solutions do not generate billions of dollars each year. This parallels the natural health science approach versus conventional medicine and drugs.

We are told crops will die without pesticides. *We,* unfortunately, will die *with* pesticides. The book *Silent Spring* warned us thirty years ago that if we don't change our ways the human race will suffer extinction.

In order to have a safe, nutritious food supply we must support farmers in producing safe and ORGANIC foods, thereby reducing carcinogens and poisons being pumped into the air, soil, and water. As Margaret Mead, anthropologist, said -- "Never doubt that a small group of committed, thoughtful citizens can change the world. Indeed, it's the only thing that ever has." When enough people care things will change.

One of the purposes of life is to improve life on Earth. We must support farmers in producing safe, economical foods for our benefit and that of future generations. Organic food is a solution.

If the produce brokers, the middlemen of agribusiness, demand safe food then we'll get it. If we as consumers demand it, the brokers will demand it from suppliers, and the farmers will supply (grow) it. We have to change the direction of the giant agricultural industry. Pretending that all is well does not, of course, make it that way.

We must ask for biological controls to be developed and used, to replace chemicals.

Society is addicted to science and technology. Science is not God, and doctors are not gods. Science and doctors basically serve greedy industries. How, then, can science and doctors be trusted to help us? We must

16

demand that doctors and science serve our interests, not theirs.

How? Follow the lead of grocery store customers, who must complain to store managers and owners. And take their business elsewhere if necessary.

Deception and manipulation are facts of life. We cannot escape it because it is human nature. So, we have met the enemy, and the enemy is us. We are our own worst enemy. Therefore, the only solution is no more chemical pesticides, no more toxic chemicals, (including pharmaceutical drugs that have not proven themselves to be nurturing or lifesaving), in our environment. Feeding ourselves poison, drinking poison, breathing poison, is slow suicide for those who are knowledgeable. For our children, and others not knowledgeable, it is murder. We *do* have a responsibility. Think about it.

* * * * *

Agricultural pesticide use is up 170% in the last eighteen years. There is a strong correlation between exposure to pesticides and cancer, which now strikes one in three Americans. "The government wants to manage cancer, not prevent it," says Michael Colby, Executive Director of Food and Water. This group has taken a stand against pesticides, seeking to develop local food safety groups called "Neighborhood Networks," and to pressure the nation's leading supermarkets and companies to provide pesticide-free products. They can be reached at 1-800-EAT-SAFE.

This organization has successfully led the fight against food irradiation for seven years. In their literature they say, "Food should give us nutrition, not cancer. Together, we will stop toxic pesticides." And, "Our health is being jeopardized by the industries that stand to gain *billions* from pesticide use, and by a government that is failing to protect consumers."

The Bible says that the land should lie fallow every seven years, to replenish its depleted nutrients. This, of course, has never been done. Instead of government subsidies/supplements for farmers -- which is really welfare -- or, government buying surplus and throwing it away, the government could support the farmer once each seven years.

* * * * *

Louisiana is first in the nation for the total amount of toxic material released into the air, water, and soil each year. Industry generates over 18 billion pounds of hazardous wastes each year, more than any other state. Louisiana imports over 800 million pounds of hazardous waste yearly. At least 40% of the lakes, rivers, and streams in that state are too contaminated for swimming, fishing, or drinking. It has three of the four largest commercial hazardous waste landfills in the country. Over 5,000 wells in the state have been used for water injection of industrial pollutants, 218.5 million pounds according to the EPA.

Figures for 1991 were: 458 million pounds of toxic chemicals, 48 million pounds greater than the second ranked state, Texas; and twice the emissions of the third ranked state, Tennessee. Louisiana discharges about 161,000 pounds of toxic chemicals into surface water, 16

18

times the amount discharged by the second largest discharger, California.

Louisiana's environmental problems and lack of responsibility seriously affect the rest of the United States. Politicians and industry leaders continue to deny it. Continue to deny the magnitude of these poisons and the death and suffering they create. This *laissez faire* attitude permeates the social structure and attitudes of the Louisiana population. A policy of non-intervention, of non-interference -- "let it be." I have lived in Louisiana for three years, and as an outsider looking in, am painfully aware the necessary changes may never happen. Apathy is not an answer.

Metropolitan Life Insurance rates Louisiana as the nation's leader in cancer mortality rates among white males, and near the top in *all* disease categories.

The deplorable situation in Louisiana motivated me to research extensively the connection between our environment and health, or the lack of it.

(The figures used here are from The Louisiana Environmental Action Network and the EPA.)

* * * * *

You can't be poisoned into health with drugs called medicines. Medicine is a commercially perpetrated myth. All so-called medicines are poisons so dangerous they are controlled substances. They can inflict permanent injury and death. Approximately 140,000 people die each year because of drug overdose in hospitals nationwide. So-called medicines have the power to destroy, but absolutely no health-giving properties. Billions of dollars a year are spent in the search for chemically derived health, by persons buying pills called medicine. In 1976, Mr.Illich, in

Limits to Medicine stated, "Doctors effectiveness is an illusion, much medical treatment is useless". And "Doctors inflict injuries on defenseless patients". Twenty years later it's still true.

Drastic operations bring in so much money that many doctors and hospitals would face economic ruin without them. Operations like heart bypass surgery, cancer operations like mastectomies and hysterectomies -- half of which doctors themselves admit are unnecessary!

America's largest industry today is the disease industry. Even criminal behavior and overweight are now called "diseases"! This industry takes at least $900 BILLION annually from the American people. Sickness is BIG BUSINESS!

The drug industry is dependent on a disease industry. The disease industry is dependent on a drug industry.

At the 15th anniversary dinner of The British Medical Association Prince Charles said, "It is frightening how dependent on drugs we are all becoming and how easy it is for doctors to prescribe them as the universal panacea for ills." The Royal Family uses homeopathic doctors.

* * * * *

There is no denying some drugs are necessary, and definite life savers. However, there needs to be more responsible and discriminating attitudes in prescribing and using drugs.

A case in point is salicylate acid, better known as aspirin. A five year government delay in requiring warning labels on aspirin led to the needless deaths of 1,470 children from Reye's Syndrome.

Two examples of side effects from prescription drugs are that about 61,000 cases of drug-induced Parkinson's disease develop yearly, and about 243,000 hospitalizations a year are necessary because of drug reactions. Also, sexual disinterest and impotence can be caused by prescription drugs.

There are also drug-induced reactions that resemble Alzheimer's. A faulty diagnosis would cause unnecessary heartache and faulty treatment.

Medical drugs interfere with body healing processes. They suppress symptoms. They are poisons, labeled accordingly. How can poisons make you healthy?

We need body-builders, not body breakers. Overuse or longterm use of any drug will cause problems, usually as a result of debilitating our immune system. Often, the effect of overuse, or longterm use, of antibiotics becomes apparent as depression, fatigue or diarrhea.

Antibiotics create mutation and resistance of bad bacteria. This includes antibiotics in meat. The end result is repeated infections, weakening of the immune system, upset enzyme balance causing poor absorption of nutrients, which further weakens the immune system.

In 1993, 70,000 Americans died as a result of hospital-acquired, anti-biotic resistant infections. The CDC in Atlanta said, "It is probably the number one public health issue. "

The epidemic of death and suffering caused by prescription drugs and medical procedures is called Iatrogenic Diseases. Can you believe it? More new "diseases" that are man-made.

According to the Journal of the American Medical Association, you have up to a 67% chance of misdiagnosis in a United States hospital today.

21

This may or may not be connected: More heart specialists die of heart attacks and strokes than the general populace.

New "diseases" seem to pop up endlessly. It is obvious research institutions, doctors, private interests, and government agencies profit hugely from these developments. Who or what does the Center for Disease Control really represent? Are old diseases introduced as new diseases, with new and frightening names, with dire implications of suffering and death? The obvious purpose would be to increase the monetary intake of the medical system, especially the pharmaceutical and research industries. Medical scares, properly promoted, are lucrative.

* * * * *

Surgery, radiation, and chemotherapy, and prescription drugs are not always mighty saviors. Safer and painless therapies are used throughout the world. These therapies include herbs, minerals and vitamins, enzymes and other supplements, nutrition in general, exercise, acupuncture, and alternative therapies like chelation therapy. These low cost, natural treatments are far less risky, less expensive, and less traumatic to the patient.

Who wants to keep you in the dark? The AMA, the FDA, physicians, self-interest groups, pharmaceutical and drug cartels, and lobbyists. The reason, of course, is power and profit. The almighty dollar. Or, should I say the almighty millions and billions of dollars.

As an example, the FDA won't recognize or endorse any procedures that don't involve synthetic drugs. This is one answer to many questions you may have about the obscurity and lack of endorsement of natural health approaches.

There are often alternatives to unsafe or dangerous medical practices. Remember, doctors are only "practicing" medicine their entire careers, and each patient is a possible victim of mistakes. Of course, it would help if they would do their jobs better. But why should they? After all, patients must pay huge fees no matter what the results. Medical doctors don't guarantee anything. And yet, they are among the wealthiest sector of society. Doctors pretend to be authority figures because of arrogance and greed. And because people meekly accept it.

*****

What Doctors Don't Tell You is a British newsletter, published since 1988, that investigates the sham science behind many medical practices. It has reported that:

-- There is a higher rate of bone fractures among the elderly in cities with fluoridated water, showing a link between brittle bones and fluoridated water.

-- "Silver" fillings are about 50% mercury, which is more toxic than lead. More than *12,000* papers have been published on the dangers of mercury fillings. It might be a reason for Alzheimer's and Multiple Sclerosis, and other health problems.

-- Pain killing drugs cause stomach bleeding -- about 200,000 cases each year. The FDA estimates these drugs kill 10,000 to 20,000 people yearly, and cause ulcers.

23

-- Researchers around the world have traced arthritis to immune system problems.

-- About 58 million people have high blood pressure. Hypertensive drugs increase mortality rates in women by 26%.

-- About 10% of all hospital admissions in the U.S. are due to adverse reactions to prescription drugs. Women are twice as likely as men to suffer adverse reactions.

-- You have about a 10% risk of catching hepatitis from donated blood. Also, it is possible to be given the wrong blood. So, donate your own blood a month before surgery.

-- About one AIDS victim out of ten doesn't show positive on blood tests. So donated blood isn't always safe.

-- Epidurals during childbirth can leave mothers with permanent backaches or headaches.

-- More people die in unnecessary surgery than in auto accidents.

-- Angioplasty is dangerous and has to be repeated. Two of 100 undergoing the procedure die on the operating table.

-- The benefits of taking hormone replacement are false.

-- The "1990 Harvard Medical Practice Study" said that three times as many Americans die from doctor's mistakes as from guns (about 100,000 a year).

-- Radical breast surgery doesn't improve chances of survival.

-- 30% of women who have hysterectomies never have sex again; 30% become infected as a result of surgery. Four out of five hysterectomies are not needed. 40% have long term depression.

-- Diet cures hyperactivity in children in about half the cases.

-- Medical tests are often expensive medical rip-offs that don't work.

-- Pap smears haven't reduced deaths from cervical cancer. The test is wrong about 60% of the time.

-- The DPT baby vaccine causes about 1000 crib deaths a year. About 50% of whooping cough victims have had vaccinations (DPT) already.

-- Doctors laugh at safe, cheap alternatives and try to have them outlawed.

-- Millions of Americans suffer from diseases and injuries doctors cause because of arrogance, stupidity and mistakes. One wrong opinion, one mistake, can devastate your life.

*****

25

Modern medicine and science have not proven themselves to be the ultimate weapon with which to fight human illness. The human being is not just a biological subject. We are physical, spiritual, and mental.

According to many doctors, present cancer treatments are a qualified failure. Time, effort, and huge expenditures of suffering and money have resulted in little gain. Except to the income of doctors and scientists. Funded by your tax dollars, The American Cancer Society was established in 1913 to eliminate cancer within 7 years. Now, more than 80 years later, it is the richest "non-profit" charity in the world. But there are *many*, many more people dying of cancer today than in 1913. And *millions* since 1913. And more kinds of cancer. One can easily guess why The American Cancer Society has hidden, or not acknowledged, the ways to cure cancer.

The foundation of today's conventional medical treatment is surgery (cutting), x-rays (burning), radiation (burning), drugs (poisons/chemicals). Failure, suffering, weakness, and death are often the result. Fact: 60 years of treating the disease instead of the patient has proven to be a failure. Fact: Degenerative diseases have increased greatly in the last 20 to 30 years. Fact: *Billions* of dollars are given yearly to research scientists and medical doctors to find cures, etc., for these diseases. None have been found. What a gigantic waste of taxpayer's money! And voluntary contributions.

The medical business is BIG Business. Businesses exist to make money. Do not be deceived.

Physicians support the pharmaceutical industry and perpetuate the poisoning of America. The drugging of America! Do not be deceived! For the most part, physicians are not philanthropists or altruists. Maybe they were in the past, but no longer. Many of them are in it for the eventual and inevitable money, the prestige, the wealth. If this were not so, their outrageous fees would instead reflect their concern for humanity by being lower - *much* lower. How many years does it take to pay back the loan sources for their 4 to 8 years of medical school? Doctors seem to think like this – "I went to medical school (a sacrifice), so my patients are going to pay dearly for my sacrifice for the rest of my life or career." Or, "I'm better than (or smarter than) the rest of humanity," etc., etc.

The arrogance of doctors and the medical establishment has bankrupted or destituted many a family. Doctors are supposed to alleviate suffering, not cause it.

Why is there a huge increase in breast cancer? Perhaps a depressed genetic ability to resist it, to resist the thousands of carcinogenic exposures we all encounter. Not a genetic predisposition to cancer, but a depressed genetic resistance, or destroyed genetic resistance. A weakening of our natural ability to resist because of increasingly debilitating lifestyles, and environment.

Once again, increased suffering and death is making the medical community more rich. Increasing sickness correlates with increasing wealth for chemical producers, pharmaceutical concerns, doctors, hospitals, researchers, etc.

Public safety laws are compromised by commercial interests. Chemical manufacturers lobby successfully against banning chemical additives. The end result is thousands of chemicals in our food and meat, many of which are proven carcinogens, in violation of the Delaney Law enacted to protect public safety.

The EPA recognizes 15 foods that have the highest levels of toxic residues of agricultural chemicals. These, therefore, have the greatest risk of causing cancer and other health problems. They are, in order of risk: tomatoes, beef, potatoes, oranges, lettuce, apples, peaches, pork, wheat, soy beans, green beans, carrots, chicken, corn, and grapes.

It is obvious organic food is a necessity for survival. If we eliminate, instead, that food which has become dangerous to eat, soon we will have to eliminate most or all food because chemicals will be allowed to proliferate endlessly. Acceptance is not the answer. Changing the system is. If enough people demand organically grown food, we'll get it. But how many are enough?

What about getting these foods from other countries? Often, they have no regulations or do not enforce them. Also, they use chemicals our companies sell to them that can't be used here, that are banned in the United States.

These unethical and immoral exchanges produce money (profit) for a few, and sickness and suffering for many.

*****

Our agricultural system is out of balance, and has been for a long time, because of using fumigants, pesticides, and fertilizers to excess. Plants, therefore, don't produce safe, nutritious food. When these plants are sick, so are we. Less nutrition can mean more cancer. New killer diseases are clear signs that our bodies are as weak as the soil. We, like all life, have a dependency on a balanced system.

DDT was banned twenty years ago in the USA because it was killing us and wildlife. Did you know pesticide companies continued to sell DDT and other USA banned toxic chemicals to third world countries? Eventually, this affects everyone.

The consumer expects the farmer will produce safe, economical food to eat. But these consumer expectations have absolutely no impact on the farmer if they don't tell him. He needs to make money, and the consumers have not communicated their needs to him. We, as consumers, must demand safe and nutritious food, free of poisons, and then buy only that kind of food. If we don't, farmers will continue to support the chemical companies by buying and using many tons of chemicals/poisons to increase yield (i.e. income) and we will be slowly destroyed by exotic diseases, mutating cancers, polluted waters, air and food. Consumers buy, and then create a demand. No demand = no product perpetuation.

If toxic chemicals continue to pollute the Earth our health dilemma is insolvable.

The FDA, the EPA, the CFA, spend billions of tax dollars to regulate and investigate the symptoms, not the causes. A lot of government programs are like pharmaceutical drugs -- they attack the symptoms not the causes of the problems.

Law enforcement is often ineffective at all levels. Laws are broken, bent and ignored. Loopholes are found, created, and used. This includes the Environmental Protection Agency and the Government.

Recently the FDA attempted to require a prescription to buy food supplements. Obviously the medical establishment is threatened by vitamins and minerals.

The American Medical Association and physicians, the Federal government and state governments, the pharmaceutical industry and insurance industry, all have vested interests in the perpetuation of disease and suffering.   What are the effects of the poisoning of America? Sickness, suffering and death for the masses. And monetary riches for the pharmaceutical and chemical industries, for physicians and insurance companies.

Hospitals are a profit motivated industry. Big Business. Do you doubt it ?

A case in point is: In 1987 a study of 500,000 (yes, *500,000*) patients concluded that indigent patients were three times more likely than insured patients to die in the hospital. Money talks.

It is logical to think health care has high standards because it costs so much. But of course it isn't so. Hospital mistakes, nurse mistakes, and doctor mistakes cause suffering and pain, and kill. Everyone can probably relate indirectly or directly to this. Unfortunately.

Eight out of ten doctors admit to ordering unnecessary and costly tests to protect themselves in case of litigation. You pay for these extra tests which are *their* safety nets.

Greed, money, power, and politics have created a world of suffering and pain and death in the part of life called "health," or the lack of health. As my grandmother would say, "If you've got your health you've got everything." Too many people don't have it.

Rachel Carson's book *Silent Spring* courageously exposed an ugly likely case scenario about thirty years ago. Apparently, national support for her ideas did not greatly influence politicians, corporations, industries, and "scientists" that pollute our life.

Do we really live in a democracy? I think it's a modified democracy, not "by the people and for the people" but by and for the politicians; the wealthy (corporate America, the insurance industry, lawyers, doctors, and the medical industry); the criminal (many

30

laws protect the criminal not the victim); and the white male (especially in the South).

"A government that withholds essential information is no more a democracy than one that speaks falsely."

-- Scott Peck, M.D.
A Road Less Traveled.

* * * * *

Each year 125,092,188 pounds of hazardous waste fuels are shipped into Louisiana, the most chemically affected state in the U.S. The second is Texas. Nearly 500,000 vehicles a year transport this on its highways. The immense danger is obvious.

The poisoning of America is in the air, the water, the soil. Recently, fish caught near an isolated island in Lake Superior contained pesticides used in tobacco planting in the southeastern U.S. It is an <u>airborne</u> pesticide. Lake Superior is regarded as the cleanest, most pure lake in the U.S. Not clean, but the *most* clean. This should leave no doubt as to the vulnerability of the world, not just the U.S. alone.

Water covers three-fourths of the Earth's surface and is one of the most basic elements of life. An absolute necessity for living. Yet, more than 98 pesticides have been allowed to contaminate our ground water in 48 states, contaminating the drinking water of more than 10 million people. This is according to a 1991 report by the General Accounting Office (GAO). So, by now, five years later, it's probably considerably worse. Are *you* one of those more than 10 million people?

The Federal government and state governments have vested interests in the perpetuation of the use of poisons. Affecting all our lives. Billions of tons of chemicals, pesticides, herbicides, nuclear wastes, radioactive wastes -- the list goes on and on.

We can't escape it, we can't seem to change it. We are victims, then, of greed, stupidity, and selfishness.

* * * * *

Every year 5 to 10 million poisonings are reported because of accidental exposures to poisons in the home. Poisons are in paint, adhesives, furniture, carpets, deodorizers, pesticides, drapes, synthetic fiber clothes, perfumes and colognes.

Persons who are repeatedly exposed to chemicals may become "saturated," developing severe reactions to anything chemical. Most building materials and their components are potentially dangerous, so we are all at risk, everyday in a way we cannot avoid. If you are unable to determine the cause of any sickness or health problem examine your home and workplace.

Complaints such as allergies, chronic fatigue, chronic sinus congestion, depression, gastrointestinal upsets, headaches, joint and muscle pain, hypertension, asthma, edema, skin rashes, mood swings, and muscle weakness can be because of toxic overloads.

When chemicals interact, the results can be *increased* toxicity. Some of us are walking chemical factories.

The U.S. produces at least 400 *billion* pounds of synthetic organic chemicals yearly. The EPA lists more than *48,000* chemicals used in the United States.

32

What does the Environmental Protection Agency do to "protect" us from these more than 48,000 poisons?

When a doctor prescribes a medicine (drug) for you, look it up in the *Physician's Desk Reference* at the public library -- you may not be willing to take it.

Environmental toxins and chemical pollutants (like smoke) cause direct irritation of tissue and cells, a weakened immune system, disruption of cellular integrity, mutation of cells due to alteration of DNA or genetic material, and altered cell structure and replication. Obviously, the significance of exposure is immense.

The average American consumes 150 pounds of food additives annually. More than 15,000 chemicals are involved in food processing and production. The chemical industry sells more than FOUR BILLION DOLLARS *yearly* of food additives.

Every year chemical companies, agricultural industries, and factories put millions of tons of pollution -- poison -- into our rivers, lakes, streams, and oceans, into the air, into the soil. If you did not buy their products, or objected to this poisoning in another effective manner, these multi-million dollar industries would not do it.

In 1962, Rachel Carson's book *Silent Spring* alerted us to the death and destruction caused by pesticides. (In fact, in 1966 she died of breast cancer.) Few took notice, few took action. The situation has now been compounded immensely because of greed, politics, and many more sources and types of poison, etc. What are you, as an individual, doing to stop this manipulation?

We must have pure food, pure water, and pure air to be healthy. Filtered water and filtered air might be the only answers to this dilemma. This is a sad reflection on the selfishness of humanity.

33

It is no longer survival of the fittest but survival of the least exposed, the most insulated, the most resistant.

Don't be a victim. Control your life and your destiny. Influence the destiny of others you love. Without pressure and spending influence, natural solutions to cancers and other diseases and sicknesses will not be promoted, will not be revealed. Natural solutions are not profitable for doctors and hospitals, or clinics. Chemical and pharmaceutical companies would lose many billions of dollars.

In the USA the drug industry is extremely powerful, and hinders and obstructs alternative medical approaches that are attempting to help people in a more natural manner. Forbidding to practice, and threats of prison sentences, are their tactics. It is almost unbelievable this can happen. Pharmaceutical industries and physicians are Big Business. Do not be deceived.

For more than 20 years *billions* of dollars have been given every year to doctors, researchers, and scientists for cancer research. Deaths from cancer have almost doubled during and since that time. This has been, and still is, a hideous waste of taxpayer's money.

There is no doubt that chemicals cause disease and suffering. The U.S. Government has given many *millions* of dollars to one man alone -- Dr. Schonwalder at Research Triangle Park, North Carolina. He uses these millions of dollars, supposedly, to "promote understanding of how chemicals and physical agents cause pathological changes that manifest as diseases". This is from the Federal Catalog of Domestic Assistance.

Why aren't many millions of dollars given to promote understanding and awareness of achieving true, *natural* health, and of how suffering and disease are caused by man's lifestyle, by big business, by big government? Greed, money, power, and vested interests are the answer. Once again.

The Hippocratic Oath states:

" I will prescribe regimen for the good of my patients according to my ability and my judgment and *never do harm* to anyone. To please no one will I prescribe a deadly drug . . . "

* * * * *

CHAPTER III
PREVENTION IS BETTER THAN CURE

Our energy requirements would probably fall 25% to 35% in an ecologically oriented economy. This would reduce our import needs for oil by more than 50%. The foods to which we are biologically adapted require less than one-tenth of the labor, energy, and resources to produce as do our present pathological foods.

You can vote for the kind of world you want with your dollars. The way you spend your money can create a better world. Don't buy health-destroying and ecologically destructive products. Push for organically produced vegetables and fruits. Support those farmers who raise organic produce and ask your grocer to get a supplier. Ask him how much of his produce is irradiated. Everything in the usual grocery store has additives, preservatives, pesticides, radiation, toxic metals, insecticides, chemicals, aluminum traces, PCB's, trans-fatty acids, etc., resulting in eventually producing health problems.

To quote Schopenauer, "With health everything is a source of pleasure; without it, nothing else is enjoyable. The greatest of all follies is to sacrifice health for any other kind of happiness, whether it be for gain, advancement, learning, or fame. Everything should be made secondary to health."

The conservation and redemption of our environment is vital to our health and that of future generations. Air, water, and land. Nothing is more important than cleaning up and purifying these elements that allow us to live.

*****

According to the *Washington Post,* an estimated 500,000 Caesarean sections are performed unnecessarily yearly. Another huge source of income is bypass surgery which, according to the American Medical Association's official journal, is performed on patients who do <u>not</u> meet the criteria for benefit about *85%* of the time.

A Harvard study revealed that in one year almost 10,000 people died in New York hospitals from doctors' mistakes, malpractice, and medical treatments. Another Harvard study showed 84% of heart patients told to have bypass surgery were found to *not* need it. Every year 17,500 patients die from this operation. Therefore, between 14,000 and 15,000 lives could be saved by better diagnosis, alternatives, better surgery, etc.

Dr. Arnold Relman, past Editor of the *New England Journal of Medicine,* said, "Patients can no longer count on their physicians to put their welfare first." In fact, doctor's fees, hospital charges, and drug prices have been the fastest rising prices on the Consumer Price Index.

A U.S. Office of Technology assessment revealed *80%* of conventional medicine has no scientific basis at all.

Enlarged prostate affects 75% of all men over fifty. Surgical removal of the prostate is common. Conventional medicine pushes Proscar®, which has been proven repeatedly to be of dubious value. However, the herb sawtooth palmetto is very effective, and safer. And cheaper. Also, zinc and flaxseed oil can be very effective.

A Harvard study revealed that kidney stones can be prevented with magnesium and vitamin B6. Too much protein causes kidney failure.

Gum disease can be eliminated simply. The bacteria primarily responsible is destroyed and placque is removed by brushing with baking soda and hydrogen peroxide.

It has been estimated that medical mistakes kill about 186,000 Americans a year. Maintaining good health, and preventing disease and mistakes are more possible if you take charge of your own health, and investigate alternatives.

Probably every adult uses under-arm deodorants. Aluminum is in 99% of deodorants/anti-perspirants. Could aluminum, or another chemical ingredient in deodorants/anti-perspirants, be a cause, or a causative factor, in breast cancer? The huge increase in breast cancer logically reflects, or indicates, a common or shared reason. Men get breast cancer too.

Could Alzheimer's increasing occurrence among women and men be connected to aluminum in deodorants/anti-perspirants? It is certain that aluminum has been repeatedly found in abnormal levels in the brains of Alzheimer's victims.

To be safe on both accounts use no deodorants/anti-perspirants containing aluminum. Alternatives are hard to find, but very possibly worth the effort. In general, clear deodorants/anti-perspirants have no aluminum.

Also, the fluoride in drinking water increases the amount of aluminum leached from cookware and absorbed into any food cooked in it. So to be safe, use no aluminum cookware, and purify water. Accumulated aluminum in the body inhibits absorption of calcium into the bones. Also, avoid wrapping food in aluminum foil. Splashing rubbing alcohol under the arms is a simple alternative to the usual aluminum-containing deodorants/anti-perspirants.

A Pastor of a local church who had a colon cancer operation follows a macrobiotic diet in the hopes of avoiding a recurrence. A friend of his had made an announcement at a meeting that he was proof of the value of a natural diet. He had had a cancer operation but the cancer returned. He then followed a macrobiotic diet and caused it to disappear. After a long time he returned to his usual diet. After a while the cancer returned. After about six months he died.

* * * * *

CHAPTER IV
THE IMPORTANCE OF YOUR LIVER

Some liver problems can be seen by accumulation of water in the abdomen (distension). This is regarded as "the beerdrinker's stomach" or "beer belly" in men, and the "appearance of pregnancy" in women. This often leads to edema of feet and ankles. Benign ovarian cysts and ovarian cancer are two more conditions causing this in some women. Cancer, severe heart failure, and kidney disease are other causes. Another is overweight.

The natural health approach will probably alleviate each one of these problems. If the problem is chronic, long-term, then it may not. Or, it just may take longer to see positive results.

The gall bladder stores bile and secretes bile into the intestine to digest fat. Gallstones are secreted along with the bile and cause an obstruction. Indigestion symptoms associated with gallstones will disappear after gallbladder removal in about only three fourths of the patients. In the USA, it is estimated that 15 million people have gallstones, with two to three times the frequency in women.

To help prevent gallstones cut down on the amount of animal fats and increase the amount of fiber. This is the latest conventional medical approach.

The liver is an immensely complicated organ, second only to the brain in complexity. The most important function of the liver is its ability to break down the food we eat and turn it into energy -- carbohydrates, fat, and protein. Also, the liver gets rid of waste products; assists in absorption of fats and vitamins; assists in the manufacture and breakdown of many hormones, enzymes and proteins; neutralizes poisons; and properly channels waste products.

During fasting the blood glucose level is prevented from falling by the conversion of glycogen back into glucose. This process is largely controlled by the liver, with the help of insulin, which is a hormone that is made in the pancreas. If the liver is badly damaged the ability to control glucose concentration in the blood is often lost.

People with liver disease take longer to heal. Skin problems and abscesses indicate that toxins aren't neutralizing in the liver. A deficient liver is incapable of secreting adequate protective substances to prevent disease. When the liver and kidneys are not working properly the heart will be overworked, resulting in edema -- swollen ankles and legs.

Alcohol, tobacco, fat, and cod liver oil cause cirrhosis and necrosis (death) of liver cells. Most medications, chemicals in foods, vaccines, over-the-counter drugs (chemicals), meat, coffee, milk, sugar, white flour, and processed oils cause deterioration of the liver. Bad habits which affect the liver are excess fatigue, overcooking, overeating, and lack of exercise.

Taking care of the liver is the best way to assure good health. Other major organs depend on the liver to produce good quality blood. No cure of any disease, no true health is possible, without a well-functioning liver. Because of bad food and chemicals sometimes it is even overworked at birth, resulting in childhood diseases and sicknesses.

The liver transforms food to utilize it. If it is not functioning well food can become toxic, poisonous. The liver prevents infection, forms blood, and transforms protein and fats. It secretes bile, which digests and assimilates fats. The liver eliminates poisons (nicotines, caffeine, chemicals, pesticides, metals, food additives, etc.) The importance of a healthy, well-functioning liver is enormous.

It is interesting to note that the liver is the only part of the human body able to regenerate itself, to replace itself, if no more than two-thirds of it is damaged or removed. Amazing!

Symptoms of a malfunctioning liver are: yellow skin and eyes, dark spots on face and hands, red nose, bitter taste in mouth, bad breath, nausea, pain below the ribs on the right side, pain in right shoulder and shoulder blades, gas on left side, headaches, sleeplessness, urinate more during the night, bad digestion, constipation alternating with diarrhea, intestinal spasms, colitis, chills after eating, mineral deficiencies, pyrosis, anemia, heartburn, diabetes, hypoglycemia, ulcers, appendicitis, underweight, overweight, vision trouble, ear trouble, edema, skin trouble, glandular imbalance, menstrual problems, flat feet, adenoids, nervousness, rheumatism, hemophilia, tuberculosis, sensitivity to insect bites, sinus trouble, head colds, cancer, gallstones, sterility, impotence, and a chronic cough. At menopause the malfunctioning liver greatly accentuates troubles.

Dr.Max Gerson said in *A Cancer Therapy* that, "After the liver shows pathological changes the body is already set in motion for more serious conditions."

To heal the liver use Montmorillonite clay. It detoxifies the liver. First thing in the morning, take 1 teaspoon with one-half cup water. Wait 15 minutes before eating anything else. Do this for at least 2 weeks. Also, rosemary tea is best for the liver, along with rosemary honey as a sweetener. Honey stimulates the liver, and may be a rehabilitating factor. (Rosemary honey is best, but others may help.) Or, take 2 to 3 tablespoons lemon juice with or without honey, on an empty stomach in the morning and before going to bed, for at least 7 days. These methods will improve the way you feel after about a week. They can be alternated, and continued for up to three months, with great benefit.

Another way to heal a dysfunctional liver is with fresh lemon juice (not frozen) mixed 10% with distilled water, taken every hour, alternated with plain distilled water every half-hour. This will flush toxins and rebuild the liver, perhaps faster than other methods. Also, there are herbal combinations to help the liver.

Remember, it took years of abuse before your liver rebelled, and it will take a long time to heal. Natural healing methods are not "quick cures." True healing eliminates the cause and restores to genuine health. So be patient and you will be rewarded!

* * * * *

Two Important Rules of Health:

It takes 5-7 times the normal amount of nutrition to build and repair the body than it does to maintain it.

Nothing heals in the human body in less than three months, then add one month for every year of sickness.

CHAPTER V
FASTING AND THE BEST DIET

We must establish a healthful approach to life. Health restoration, maintenance, or achievement happens as a result of education and guidance in health issues, and adherence to the simple knowledge and necessary life approaches. We must share knowledge of health, of natural ways to end sickness and disease. Pathogenic practices must be discontinued. Internal cleansing and superior nourishment are necessary. Improper nutrition and toxicosis cause sickness and disease. Correct this problem for optimum health.

Humans are anatomically and physiologically adapted to a diet of fruits, vegetables, and nuts, and some seeds. Businesses that sell meat and milk products have entrenched interests, as does the American government, in perpetuating the myth we must have, we need to have, meat and milk. An educated population would bring an end to their niche in the marketplace, and a decrease in many diseases.

All proteins are composed of amino acids. The best sources of concentrated proteins for people are raw nuts and seeds, unsalted. They also contain all vitamins, minerals, trace elements, carbohydrates, and hormones. Apples, apricots, avocados, grapes, olives, and tomatoes are especially rich in proteins, i.e. amino acids.

There are no amino acids (protein) in flesh that the animal did not derive from the plant. When you eat *raw* fruit and vegetables you get carbohydrates, hormones, minerals, vitamins, chlorophyll, and amino acids, trace elements, and fatty acids.

44

The human stomach lacks sufficient acid for proper digestion of meat. The small intestine and colon are three times longer than carnivorous animals, so meat putrefies before expulsion. So, don't eat meat! We are frugivores (fruit eaters), not carnivores.

The body needs proper nutrition for recovery, or restoration, and maintenance. For complete health. Fresh, only raw, fruit, with some raw vegetables, nuts, and seeds, is proper nutrition. This is the Best Diet for all of us. Combined with fasting, this approach to living might be called the fountain of youth formula. It's possible to look and feel years younger in about 30 days.

*****

Raw juice (not canned or with additives) purifies blood and tissues, helps cell and tissue regeneration, restores mineral balance, and provides an alkaline surplus for restoration of health. Juice is easily assimilated and digested.

According to European Dr.Johannes Kuhl, fermented lactic acid juices (sold in health food stores) possess extraordinary medical properties for treatment of cancer, digestive disorders, kidney and liver diseases, and arthritis.

For most health problems juice made with any available green leafy vegetables from the garden (including vegetable tops) and mixed with a glass of carrot, beet, and celery juice is extremely beneficial. Lemon apple juice cleanses wastes and toxins from the body, and is good for weight loss.

When fruit and vegetables (juice or whole) are eaten together, only partial assimilation of nutrients results. And indigestion.

45

Drink juices between meals, not with meals. Drink slowly for greatest benefit. Make only as much as is needed because storage depletes value. Dilute with water if it's too sweet, or if you're diabetic or hypoglycemic.

Up to 95% of the food value is found in the rinds, seeds, peels, and stems. Some juicers can make use of these valuable nutrients. However, citrus peels and rinds, and other fruit skins, absorb all the chemicals sprayed on them. So, organically produced fruit is essential.

Freshly made juices have enzymes -- a life source. Bottled and canned juices have an extended shelf life because the enzymes have been killed. Fresh juice nutrients, however, are perfectly balanced.

Because the American diet consists of many processed "dead" foods, we are undernourished. In 1914 the United States was ranked among the most healthy countries in the world. But today we are 79th. Yes, 79th.

Fasting is the oldest therapeutic method known to man and woman. It is the best method for losing weight as well as healing. In Germany and Sweden fasting has been used to treat every disease. According to many authorities on fasting, it is the most effective healing method known to man, and the safest (when it's a raw juice, vegetable broth, and herbal tea fast, not the traditional water fast). You can feel stronger, have more vitality, and be rid of health problems. Dr.Otto Buchinger had supervised over 90,000 successful fasts. Dr.Airola had supervised hundreds of fasts with remarkable results. If you fast on your own then try to get his book, *How to Keep Slim, Healthy, and Young with Juice Fasting,* for do-it-yourself fasting.

Dr.Christian Barnard, famous heart surgeon, suffered for years from rheumatism and allergies. He said that because of fasting and a raw wholefood diet he had been able to keep his symptoms in check. Ted Danson, of the TV series *Cheers* and movie fame, said in an interview in *Gentleman's Quarterly* that he fasts for three days every month to clean out toxins.

*****

To prepare yourself for fasting, eat only raw fruits and vegetables for a few days before. After 3 to 7 days of juice, broth, and/or herbal tea fasting, break the fast by gradually working up to a normal diet. Do not overeat, eat slowly, chew well. Then continue to follow the Best Diet. After a few weeks, you may want to fast again for 3 to 7 days.

Anyone on drugs for a long time (digitalis, insulin, or cortisone in particular) should not have an unsupervised fast. Neither should very sick or very weak persons, or those with advanced diseases or diabetics. In those cases, consult your doctor.

If you fast for more than three days bowel movements usually cease. Toxic wastes are mainly eliminated through the bowels, so enemas are necessary. If these toxins remain in your colon they will be reabsorbed into the system, poisoning your whole body, or maybe overloading your kidneys.

About one third of all body impurities and wastes are expelled through the skin. Daily showers and brisk rubs with a rough towel help accomplish this.

*****

In 1943, *Scientific American* magazine reported: "Grass is high in vitamin C, beta carotene, calcium, and vitamin B. Everyone should eat it daily! " Instead, people

47

eat the cows that prosper on it. This is ultimately very harmful. Vegetarians have low blood pressure and cholesterol levels–two major risk factors for heart disease. This is attributed to not eating meat. As everyone knows, vegetarians usually live longer than meat eaters. By combining foods from various sources, it is not difficult for vegetarians to get sufficient protein, i.e. amino acids.

There are over 100,000 types of protein in the human body. If you just avoid foods of animal origin without following the proper diet you will develop deficiencies, with symptoms like hypoglycemia-- dizziness and lack of energy. Protein starvation would eventually have serious consequences. But if your body cannot digest or utilize ingested protein you can still have a deficiency even with an *excess* intake of protein.

If you want to achieve your full health potential, you must adopt the living food diet. Eat plenty of raw fruits and vegetables, plus three or four ounces of raw nuts and/or seeds daily and you will get everything you need. This is the Best Diet. The pathological effects of food cooked above 118° F include an abnormally high white corpuscle count (leukocytosis). Unprocessed grains are the best sources of fiber. Wholegrain brown rice balances the acid/alkaline level and produces a nice variation in a proper, only beneficial, diet. This is maybe the best unprocessed grain, but oats, barley, and wheat also promote a good cleansing action.

This fruit, vegetables, grain, seeds, and nuts diet is similar to a traditional Oriental diet -- significant because Orientals have about one-tenth to one-twelfth the occurrence of heart disease, osteoporosis, and cancer. Their diet is worth emulating!

"Ishoku Dogen" is an old Japanese saying that means: "Medicine and food have the same source."

* * * * *

Eating a diet high in fiber can help eliminate or avoid gallstones, colitis, appendicitis, hiatus hernia, constipation, diarrhea, hemorrhoids, varicose veins, and diabetes. It helps control diabetes by slowing the rate at which the body absorbs glucose. The function of a high fiber diet, a diet high in fruits and vegetables that are fresh and raw, is to regulate and normalize the way your body metabolizes nutrients. It provides the means to move things smoothly through the system, picking up toxins and waste, maximizing the absorption of nutrients and blocking fermentation and infection in the digestive tract. The prevention of disease is one of the results, detoxifying our bodies is another.

Fiber satisfies the appetite by giving a feeling of fullness, making it ideal for weight control. It helps prevent the recycling of liver bile because it prevents bile from being absorbed and reused. So the bile gets flushed from the body, and new bile is made. The main ingredient of bile is cholesterol, which is taken from the bloodstream. So soluble fiber lowers cholesterol.

Psyllium, in powder form, is a very beneficial dietary addition to ensure adequate fiber intake. The main cause for almost all illness is in the liver, the digestive system, or the colon. Therefore, we must take nourishment which will help get rid of waste through normal channels. High fiber in the form of psyllium, or unprocessed whole grains and organic fruits and vegetables (raw), will ensure this. Also, the first thing to encourage a cure is to secure the evacuation of organs affected. A lot of high fiber in your diet can do this, at least partly.

Refined foods have been homogenized, irradiated, separated, blanched, fermented, hydrogenated, saturated, deep fat fried, degerminated, boiled, gassed, dyed, aerated, artificialized, preserved, and packaged. *Ninety percent* of everything in grocery stores has been refined.

Most of the foods eaten today form mucous in the intestinal tract. *So does air pollution.* This mucous builds in the intestines, blocking proper elimination, and becoming a breeding ground for germs and parasites that pollute the blood and lymphs, and eventually the entire system. This causes a chronic drain on vitality and health. So it is necessary to remove this accumulation that never leaves the body of most people. This toxicity can contribute to the development of disease.

It is important to maintain a healthy population of lactobacteria in the intestinal tract to counteract harmful bacteria. Taking psyllium daily for two or three months depletes the lactobacteria in the intestines, but it is very effective at removing stagnant material. The lactobacteria need to be stimulated to multiply.

Yogurt containing lactobacillus acidophilus, or lactobacillus acidophilus tablets available at health food stores, are solutions. Fructooligosaccharides (FOS) is a class of carbohydrates found in fruits and vegetables. It dramatically increases the growth of friendly bacteria, such as lactobacillus acidophilus and bifidobacteria, in the intestines. Acidophilus is the friendly flora that prevents bad micro-organisms from settling in the gastrointestinal and genitourinary tract.

A non-mucous forming diet is obviously necessary for the success of any method to cleanse the intestinal tract. Re-introducing those foods after will cause the problem to occur again. Raw fruits and vegetables (organically grown), sprouts, grains including millet, and seeds, are the necessary food, once again, to avoid accumulation of toxicity in the intestinal tract which depletes vitality and health, and may lead to diseases like colon cancer. But how do we avoid air pollution?

* * * * *

Fasting may reverse almost all health problems except truly terminal cases and those in which irreversible organic damage has been sustained. It can make anyone look years younger, especially if you're over 40. You can purify and rejuvenate yourself. Even "incurable" health problems have been healed after fasting. Blood pressure is normalized, tumors and growths are autolyzed, stress is eliminated, cravings and addictions for alcohol, tobacco, coffee, drugs, etc., are eliminated.

The body can resolve its problems faster while fasting than in any other life mode. Fasting is the condition under which the body's remedial powers are most pronounced. The benefits of fasting, raw diet, and exercise need to be common knowledge.

After fasting, eat organic raw fruits and vegetables, seeds and nuts. It is an easy, simple, better way to eat. This diet gives energy and health. The usual United States diet is pathogenic, processed, toxic, nutrient deficient, and energy draining. The Basic Four food group is really a division of the marketplace among commercial interests. Giant food companies have dictated what we will eat on the basis of what is profitable to them. Nutritionists and dietitians, no matter how sincere, have been trained to serve commercial interests rather than our populace's health needs.

Eating this simple, easy way would solve many complex environmental problems. As an example, we

51

have polluted our water so badly that in many cases fish are no longer able to spawn in our rivers, lakes, streams, and oceans. Eliminate the many tons of chemicals poured into them yearly and they will begin a process of self-recovery, with our assistance and help. Organically produced food is part of the solution.

If you eliminate chemicals/poisons you'll eliminate many allergies. In fact, eliminate chemicals/poisons to eliminate *many*, many health problems. But be patient. Without fasting as a precursor to this change (and even with fasting) years of exposure to these dangers cannot be undone in a few days. Persevere and you will be rewarded! Remember, it may take weeks or months to undo the damage inflicted on your body, but improvement is inevitable, unless irreversible organic damage has been sustained.

The actual healing process will only start after neutralization of the blood. The detoxification process must be slow so that a strain on the system is avoided. The idea, "The steady drop hollows the stone" applies here. Therefore, a modified dietary change may be preferable, and is definitely easier. One meal a day for a while, then two, then three meals. Any moderation delays benefit, however, and invites failure and disappointment. But any improvement is better than none!

Before treatment of any health problem begins, detoxification must take place to enable an effective cure. Fasting, or modified fasting, is imperative. Fluids cleanse the body and dispose of waste material. The importance of this cannot be overemphasized. Filtered water and pure fruit and/or vegetable juice are necessary for fasting, or otherwise.

Balance and harmony are gone when any disease is present. Therefore, restore balance and harmony to affect a cure. This is only logical, and it works! There is a cause for every effect, and an effect for every cause.

* * * * *

Fasting is necessary to help heal and to throw off parasites, diseases, growths, mucous, poisonous toxins, tumors, etc. Exercise is necessary to move this through the lymphatic system.

Modified fasts take longer but are easier to endure. No hunger pains, no craving for foods. Try only apple juice for three days. The next time try it for seven days. Or, try one fruit for three days, then seven days at a later date. Or, try an all watermelon diet for ten days. This clears up health problems, makes you look years younger, gives energy, cleanses out impurities. And you'll lose weight.

For some people fasting for longer than two days may cause complications of existing problems. However, chronic, pathological conditions can be reversed through fasting. Thousands of documented cases have proven this to be so.

A major proponent of fasting is T. C. Frye. He has written many books, etc. on the subject. He has operated a wellness retreat in California for many years with a high success rate. According to him, and many other advocates of this lifestyle approach, exercise, raw diet, adequate sleep, and occasional fasting have reversed arthritis, adult onset diabetes (on insulin less than three years), asthma, psoriasis, heart problems, acne, allergies, insomnia, backache, headaches, high blood pressure, indigestion, gallbladder and liver problems, and other problems deemed incurable. Hundreds of testimonials support this lifestyle and curative approach. Harvey and Marilyn Diamond, authors of the best-selling *Fit for Life*, were students of T.C. Frye.

*****

Our diet is determined by our biological adaptations. Humans are a class of animals called frugivores. Raw fruit is the right thing to eat. Cooked fruit (and any other food) results in health problems. Cooking destroys foods by destroying nutrients. The deranged products of cooking are pathogenic leukocytosis, which occurs after eating foods that have been cooked. Fresh fruit and vegetables that are raw are easier to digest, requiring little digestive action. They are complete -- providing calories, proteins (amino acids), vitamins, minerals, and other food factors necessary to health. Our natural diet is fruits, but we can benefit from vegetables, nuts, grain, and seeds. As an example, whole grain cereal and bread, dried apricots and raisins, are high in iron. Enzymes in raw food help cause digestion, nerve impulses, detoxification, DNA and RNA, repairing, healing, thinking, memory, and the making of all hormones.

Proteins and starches should not be eaten together because proteins require an acid medium for digestion, and starches require an alkaline medium. Combining them results in indigestion. The American diet is an indigestion factory!

Dairy products cannot be digested well, because after age three the enzyme rennin ceases to be secreted by humans. Also, few adults produce lactase, necessary to digest lactose found in milk and other dairy products. Therefore, almost everyone over age three has a lactose intolerance!   It is *not* a medical problem or health deficiency.

Pasteurization destroys enzymes, amino acids, and vitamins, causing excess mucous in the body. So dairy products should be made from raw milk only. Since this is almost impossible, eliminate dairy products from your diet. Very little calcium is actually derived from milk that is pasteurized. This unnatural calcium is deposited in the arteries and may contribute to hardening of the arteries.

Animal protein, white sugar, and white flour slow down the cleansing process. This forms mucous which the body must work hard to eliminate. Excess mucous may lead to diseases like colon cancer, etc.

The body needs fats, but only use cold-pressed olive oil, cold- pressed flax oil, or raw butter. For sweeteners, use only raw honey, or pure maple syrup. Farm eggs are more nutritious and easily assimilated because they come from a more humane source. Factory eggs are produced under very cruel conditions.

Cold-pressed olive oil is the most healthy type of fat, along with cold-pressed flaxseed oil. Its cholesterol is completely different from the dangerous cholesterol obtained by eating the flesh of animals. Both these oils are of great benefit to the intestines and the liver.

Temperatures in excess of 118° F damage the quality, destroy enzymatic activity, and reduce or eliminate nutrient value of all foods. That's why oils must be cold-pressed, why fruit and vegetables should be raw. That's why hydrogenated, pasteurized (high heat processed) dairy products harm, but raw dairy products do not. When oils are heated carcinogenic substances are produced.

For better health, supplement your daily diet with cottage cheese and flaxseed oil. Dr. Johanna Budwig has been nominated seven times for the Nobel Prize for her discoveries of the benefits of eating cold-pressed flaxseed oil blended with low fat cottage cheese. Flaxseed oil is nature's best source of linolenic and linoleic acid -- the essential fatty acids -- which have been processed out of most U.S. foods. Use 2 tablespoons oil, plus one quarter cup cottage cheese daily. With this, she has restored health for hopeless cases. Truly remarkable!

* * * * *

More than 2000 years ago, we were told to eat fruit predominately, and use leaves, i.e. herbs and plants, for medicine. In the Bible, in Ezekiel, it says: "The fruit of the tree is for man's meat, and the leaves are for man's medicine."

Dr.Max Gerson, whom Dr. Albert Schweitzer called "one of the most eminent scientists in medical history", said that cancer develops because of a poisoned liver. He thought the poisons originate from chemicals in air, food, and water, and nutritional deficiencies (which poison cells). Dr.Gerson recommended in <u>1946</u> that only organic, natural food should be eaten. Why was this ignored? *Many billions* of dollars have been spent in the interim of fifty years on research. *Millions* of people have suffered. Perhaps it is apparent to you that disease and suffering are "Big Business."

Phytochemicals are natural chemical compounds found in *all* plants. Some have powerful disease prevention capabilities. Phytochemicals are the ingredients in herbs that give them their healing and therapeutic powers. They are anti-carcinogenic, anti-mutagenic, anti-oxidative and anti-inflammatory. There are approximately ten times more phytochemicals in

56

whole (raw) foods -- fruit and vegetables -- than in extracted juice.

The former U.S. Surgeon General said that 66% of all deaths in the U.S. are diet related.

We can, indeed, live nearly poison-free in this very poisoned world. The benefits of fasting, raw foods, and exercise are easily proven by anyone. Achieve health through healthful practices, including fresh air, sunshine, pure water, and adequate sleep. (Proper blood circulation is greatly helped by adequate and comfortable sleep.) And, of course, organically grown raw fruits and vegetables, seeds, and nuts are necessary for true and lasting health.

* * * * *

Studies have shown that athletes that are mainly vegetarian have twice as much endurance as meat eating athletes.

Your heart is the most responsive organ to nutritional therapy. A diet high in citrus fruit, other fruit, and vegetables reduces heart disease and strokes. Dairy products, meat, white flour and processed foods cause fatty deposits in arteries, blocking blood flow to the heart and brain. These foods, including hydrogenated oils, cause heart attacks and strokes. We are killing ourselves slowly by eating meat and processed food.

A common problem the Best Diet can overcome is stomach ulcers. This shows itself as a burning sensation in the throat, starting from the stomach. Or, belching that burns the throat, caused by acid liquid. This is caused by defective sugar metabolism, or an insufficient secretion of bile. Aloe vera and cold-pressed oils are also very helpful.

Nutritional problems can mimic far more dangerous illnesses. Less than one-half of 1% of United

States doctors have a basic knowledge of nutrition. No wonder they rely on drugs and surgery. Nutritional and natural approaches to healing are safer, simpler, cheaper, and often more effective.

Another benefit of adopting the Best Diet approach is loss of weight -- slow, gradual, and permanent weight loss without hunger or calorie counting. Then, automatic regulation and stabilization of optimum individual weight level. Loss of aches and pains, and energy increase are other benefits.

Ultimately, you will feel better. Eventually, when you break this diet routine and indulge in some food you used to crave, or just greatly enjoyed, you may find your digestive system rebelling, or your allergy reactions returning. Probably in a modified manner. This is a sure sign of the importance of continuing your Best Diet routine. This is a signal to alert you to the foods to avoid. These are part of the answer, then, to the source of your physiological imbalance.

Raw fruit and vegetables, seeds, and nuts, immediately release enzymes, breaking down food for absorption and digestion. Cooked food above 118° F has no enzymes to do this because the enzymes are destroyed. Degenerative diseases may originate from enzyme deficiencies. Digestive enzymes, then, increase absorption of food. Fruits rich in enzymes are bananas, avocados, and mangoes.

* * * * *

Hippocrates said, "Our food should be our medicine, our medicine should be our food." Garlic, lemon, sunflower seeds, organically grown fruits and vegetables, flaxseed oil, brewer's yeast, and kelp especially fulfill this need.

Both Carl Jung and Sigmund Freud predicted physiological therapy, including nutrition, would eventually prove to be more effective in helping mental illness than psychotherapy. As an example, EFA's (essential fatty acids) and brewer's yeast can eliminate depression. Also, kelp is very helpful for low thyroid and consequent depression. In the Orient, kelp is thought to enhance health, longevity, and happiness.

Flax oil is one of the richest sources of valuable Omega-3 fatty acid, having almost twice as much as do fish oils. Omega-3 dissolves tumors, and slows down our bodies' production of toxic biochemicals, providing calmness under stress. Dr. Johanna Budwig in Germany has documented over a thousand cases of successful cancer treatment using fresh, cold-pressed flax oil and nutritional support, for over 30 years. Because nausea can result from exceeding the liver's capacity for fats and oils, start with one teaspoon. Use 3 tablespoons fresh, organic flaxseed oil mixed with 7 tablespoons cottage cheese, tofu, or yogurt. Add fruit, maple syrup, honey, or vegetables and spices, for variety. This mixture will build and restore health. Many health problems can be helped or eliminated with cold-pressed flax oil supplementation.

Millet and buckwheat are the most nutritionally complete grains available. Use them as cereal.

Sunflower seeds have high percentages of zinc, EFA, vitamin D, vitamin E, calcium, and magnesium in them, and are therefore especially beneficial food -- being unprocessed, pure, and easily attainable.

A proven European remedy to restore health is fresh beetroot, which is anti-cancerous. They combine the beetroot with carrots and apples, as a salad, to eat daily for several weeks. Many thousands have benefited from its effectiveness.

For better health, eat five or six small meals a day, instead of two or three large ones. This solves low blood sugar problems (hypoglycemia), and tendency to gain weight. To improve digestion eat food groups, separately, because every group requires a different enzyme system for digestion. Combinations result in indigestion and gas. Eating less means food will be better assimilated, digested, and utilized. This means you'll feel less hungry. Eating too much actually poisons the system, especially too much protein.

Algae, harvested wild and without synthetic ingredients, is great for your health. It has vitamins, 20 amino acids, minerals, trace elements, and enzymes. It has 300% more oxygen than alfalfa. It has more protein than meat, fish, eggs, or dairy products. The results of eating it are reduced stress, increased energy and mental clarity, improved digestion, and increased immune functions.

New, healthy cells are produced to replace the diseased ones as a result of fasting. Vitamin and mineral supplements may interfere with the cleansing process -- discontinue temporarily. Herbs help cleanse and regulate, however, so try them during fasting if you want. Drink unlimited glasses of juice (without sugar) daily. Fresh juice gets 2 to 3 times more enzymes into your system in about one third the time as fresh fruits or vegetables. The first three days are the hardest to tolerate, but the most benefit comes after the third day. Toxic buildups need about three days minimum to be eliminated. An alternative is distilled water, herb teas (no sugar), and/or vegetable broths. Walk each day of the fast. Since you're eating something, this is a modified fast, and is preferably repeated the next month. Or have a grapefruit fast for 7 to 14 days to help yourself feel younger and look younger, besides ridding your body of toxins and health problems.

After a modified fast, don't eat any food that is processed, packaged, canned, or cooked. As an example, when you eat cereal eat only whole grain. Anything else is fractionated, altered, processed; deprived of its *original* natural nutrients, with chemically derived nutrients added after this depletion process. Use no lard, shortening, margarine, or vegetable oil which is hydrogenated or polyunsaturated. These are chemical processes used to extend shelf life in these harmful fats. Use only cold-pressed safflower, corn, sunflower, flaxseed, and olive oils. Margarine contains modified fat, fat molecules which produce leaky cellular membranes. Also, eating margarine greatly increases risk of cancer.

Fruit and vegetables, and green tea, have phenols and polyphenols, such as quercetin, ellagic acid, and chlorogenic acid. These help allergies, diabetes, vascular problems, infections, and reduce the risk of cancer.

*****

Digestion results in an acid residue or an alkaline residue. There must be a proper ratio between acid and alkaline foods in the diet to maintain a strong resistance to disease. In healing disease, a high alkaline balance speeds recovery. The ideal ratio is 4:1, or 80% alkaline-producing foods and 20% acid-producing foods. Acid-forming foods are seeds, nuts, and grains. Alkali-forming foods are vegetables and fruits.

The best biological treatment for many health problems is repeated short juice fasts -- juice every 2 to 4 hours for 3 to 7 days. This usually normalizes all body functions, eliminates biochemical disorder and imbalances, and restores a person to excellent health. How many fasts? As many as you need to get excellent health. The cleansing and normalizing effect of fasting on all body functions is the reason for its healing effect.

Follow this fast with a raw vegetable and fruit (peeled if not organically grown), nuts, grain, and seed diet, and you will attain and maintain superior and wonderful health. But who can eat all meals, forever, uncooked? So, try 80% uncooked, and 20% cooked. Also, who can refrain indefinitely from one's favorite (and harmful) foods? A realistic approach is to indulge occasionally, maybe as a reward for your maintenance of better health! After a while you will prefer what's good for you.

As long ago as 1968, Dr.Airola, nutritionist, said that cooked animal proteins can cause serious health disorders, and are extremely harmful when consumed in excess -- causing arthritis, kidney damage, osteoporosis, heart disease, cancer, diabetes, premature aging, lower life expectancy, etc.

Oatmeal and bran can counteract this damage by discouraging fat from clumping in blood vessels. And, fresh apples clear cholesterol from the blood. But meat must be eliminated from the diet so this can be accomplished.

John Robbins, of Baskin-Robbins fame, has written a book called *Diet For A New America*. He documents that 60 million people a year could be adequately fed by the grain saved if only Americans reduced their intake of meat by just 10%. This is equivalent to the number of people on our planet who will starve to death this year alone. A shameful reality like this needs to be changed.

Central American rainforests are the source of 40% of the world's *oxygen*. However, these forests are rapidly being destroyed to support the meat eating diet in the United States. This frightening correlation should disturb and alert everyone. Even people who insist on eating cattle need to breathe. Americans need to be informed about the consequences of their habits.

*****

Dr.Hans Selye, a famous Canadian doctor, said: "Disease and aging begin when the normal process of cell regeneration and rebuilding slow down. This is caused by the accumulation of waste products in tissues which interferes with the nourishment and oxygenation of cells". Various ills will start to appear. This can happen at any age.

At any given time, about one fourth of all your cells are in the process of dying and replacement. Fasting eliminates these and other toxic waste products that have accumulated. For this reason, it is necessary to drink juices often and exercise in some way (walking is fine), to enable the body to eliminate this toxicity, these poisons. At some point during fasting you may feel badly or your condition may worsen, because of the overload that can occur. This is temporary. Exercise and drink juice to eliminate these poisons from your body and you will feel much better than before you began the fast.

After the third day of fasting the body will burn and digest its own tissues and cells that are diseased, damaged, aged, or dead. This includes tumors, abscesses, fat deposits, and dead cells. Dr. Airola said, "This is the secret of the extraordinary effectiveness of fasting as a curative and rejuvenative therapy." Dr.Otto Buchinger, M.D., a fasting authority, called fasting "a burning of rubbish."

During a juice fast the liver, lungs, kidneys and skin pores are relieved of the usual burden of digesting food and eliminating wastes. Their cleansing capacity is increased greatly, therefore, and masses of metabolic wastes and toxins are quickly expelled. Drinking juices helps this process and the process of recovery and rejuvenation.

*****

As we age, our body's ability to assimilate or produce and synthesize chromium, CoQ10, and enzymes decreases. Therefore, various mechanisms in the body begin to malfunction, to fail, resulting in medical problems developing. Resulting in aging. As an example, chromium helps burn fat. Therefore, its decrease is a reason for a "middle age spread," that inevitable weight gain.

When there is an imbalance (sickness), create a balance with supplementation of the missing nutrients to restore health. However, to enable better utilization of these supplements, vitamin and mineral supplementation is complimentary. Remember,vitamins will not work without minerals. As a matter of fact, the beginning of any illness may be mineral deficiencies. Dr.Linus Pauling, winner of two Nobel Prizes, said "You can trace every sickness, every disease, and every ailment to a mineral deficiency." Elimination of chemicals, exercise (like walking), internal cleansing, adequate sleep, and purified water also allow the body to utilize any necessary supplements.

There are many anti-oxidants (which are cancer inhibitors), that are more powerful than vitamin A, E, C, and selenium. These are: CoQ10 (from plants and fruits), superoxide dismatuse (from alfalfa sprouts, copper and zinc), pau d'arco (from the South American lapacho tree), Essiac tea (made from 4-8 herbs), spirulina (algae) and chlorella, germanium, laetrile (from amygdalin in apricot kernels), octacosanol (from red wine and spinach), grapeseed extract, una de gato (from the cat's claw vine).

CoQ10 produces cellular energy. A deficiency of it means health problems. This has been known since the 1950's. Why hasn't it been widely recognized in the USA until recently? Millions of Japanese people have used it for many years. It is interesting to note that in the past Japanese doctors were paid for keeping people healthy, and they were not paid when people were sick.

* * * * *

Cellular destruction by free-radicals eventually breaks down the immune system and causes aging. Free-radical damage may play a role in many age-related diseases like cancer, heart disease, Parkinson's and other neurological diseases, cataracts, arthritis, graying hair, and wrinkling of the skin. Free-radical production is increased by tobacco smoke, air pollution, stress, and ultraviolet light.

Anti-oxidants are the best protection against oxygen free-radicals. All anti-oxidants prevent or slow down excessive oxidation by neutralizing free-radicals, by controlling their production, and by helping to detoxify the system. All anti-oxidants, as listed, help the immune system regenerate, so that you feel younger, look younger, and live longer.

About 1980 I read a report in a scientific magazine about two scientists in their thirties who had been testing the anti-oxidants vitamins A, C, E, and selenium on themselves for several years. Their physician reported them to be like teenagers physiologically.

Aging is caused by deficient utilization of nutrients, inadequate enzymes, and insufficient anti-oxidants to counteract increasing free-radical damage, decreased oxygen to cells, inadequate sleep, stress (emotional and physical), and increased accumulation of poisons in the intestines, liver, etc.

*****

CHAPTER VI
ECOLOGY AND HEALTH

The Earth needs our help. Simple steps can be taken to prevent pollution, protect wildlife, and preserve our natural resources for future generations, and protect ourselves from some future health problems.

Use energy efficiently -- less heat, higher air conditioner temperatures, more insulation, monitored auto trips. Don't let your car idle more than one minute.

Save water. Shut off water while brushing your teeth. Run your dishwasher and washing machine only when full. Only 3% of the water found on Earth is fresh.

Choose U.S. grown pine, oak, or cherry over tropical woods like mahogany and teak. Buy recycled paper products. Plant a tree, and support community tree planting programs. Buy rainforest products like nuts, oils, and fruits. Recycle paper. Recycling one ton of paper saves 17 trees.

Lessen garbage. Americans produce about one ton of trash, per American, per year. Only 10% is recycled. To help: *buy less, reuse and recycle.*

To reduce toxic waste, garden and landscape organically. To clear clogged drains pour in one quarter cup baking soda, followed by one half cup vinegar, and flush later with boiling water.

All this information is from EarthShare, a charitable federation of 40 non-profit environmental organizations, located in Washington, D.C.

* * * * *

The Pacific Yew tree, found in the Northwestern United States, was treated as a "trash" tree until it was found to contain taxol, an ingredient proven effective in treating cancer. What other natural sources are gone forever? There probably was, or is, a natural solution for all of Mankind's health problems.

There are several thousand plants in Costa Rican rainforests and, so far, 225 of them could produce life saving drugs. Yet, the rainforests continue to be burned. The only way to ensure survival of plant and animal species is to preserve sufficient habitat. Our survival and quality of life may depend on it.

Humanity is disrupting the natural ability of the Earth to heal itself. Humanity is disrupting the ability of itself to heal itself on an individual basis. Humanity, however, can make constructive choices to stop this destructiveness.

We need to help save the Earth. We can do this by reducing, reusing, and recycling. By preventing, protecting, and preserving. We need to help save ourselves. By preventing, protecting, and preserving ourselves and other beings.

It's all interrelated. You help one and you help the other. Save one and you save the other. You can't change society but you can change yourself.

*****

Organic food is energy producing and health building. It is estimated the average child receives four times more exposure than an adult to at least eight widely used cancer causing pesticides in food grown in the usual non-organic manner. No one knows exactly how many cases of poisonings, sicknesses and deaths are caused by pesticides yearly.

Without good soil, good plants providing optimum nutrition cannot be grown. Soil is the foundation of the food chain. With today's farming methods, topsoil is being eroded seven times faster than it is being built up. Organic farming builds and improves the soil by using green manure, human energy instead of fossil fuel, and crop covers to build the soil. Conventional farming plants the same crop year after year, robbing the soil of nutrients. This is then replaced by chemical fertilizers and makes crops more susceptible to pests, thereby perpetuating the ugly pesticide cycle.

Organic farming alleviates the *billions* of dollars in Federal agricultural subsidies (welfare for farmers); helps stop polluted water and loss of wildlife habitat; stops erosion; ends the expense of regulating and testing synthetic chemicals and monitoring their residue in foods; and (last, but not least) organic farming would eliminate the huge cost for disposal and clean-up of hazardous waste generated by pesticide manufacturers. Also, a lot of energy is used to produce synthetic fertilizers, and this fossil fuel energy would be saved.

Organic farming supports the smaller farmer. In the past decade, more than 650,000 family farms have been lost in the U.S. Two mail order suppliers of high quality organic food are: Diamond Organics at 1-800-922-2396, in Freedom, California; and Natural Lifestyle Supplies at 1-800-752-2775, at 16 Lookout Drive, Asheville, North Carolina 28804.

Organic food tastes better and looks better. Can you remember juicy, vine-ripened tomatoes being available anywhere? The symbol of modern farming is now the pale, hard, tasteless tomato.

*****

Studies have shown that criminal behavior and mental problems can be eliminated with a natural, organically produced diet. Allergies to sugar have been determined, repeatedly, to cause aberrant behavior. Hyperactive behavior can be connected to food additive allergies, and any other allergies. It is estimated that one half the U.S. population has allergies to something, somewhere. Allergies are abnormal afflictions. Pure air, pure water, and pure (organically grown, not processed) food can eliminate most of these allergies. Elimination of chemicals from your environment will probably stop other allergies that are not food connected.

To raise your energy and performance levels, and rid your body of allergy-causing toxic substances, you need to exercise daily. Walking is sufficient. Daily exercise increases your efficiency, reduces stress, improves your heart and digestion, helps your cardiovascular system, and produces a more dynamic personality. You'll need less sleep, and work more efficiently. Exercise, therefore, gives you time instead of taking it!

Children need to know they are valued to feel valuable. This is an essential aspect of mental health, and is a direct product of parental love. It can be impossible to acquire in adulthood. I know this from experience.

Being loved and appreciated is a prime need of life. Feeling good about yourself and others results from how you live. Associations with people should improve your mental, emotional, and physical well-being, not cause stress and depression. The more positive social contacts a person has the longer and healthier their lives are. Unresolved emotional stress seems to suppress immunity

70

and increases health risks like cancer and heart disease. But, laughter and good feelings that are part of social contacts provide other health bonuses -- such as lowering risks of heart disease and cancer. In fact, Norman Cousins wrote a book about how he believes laughter helped cure his cancer! Help heal disease with love and happiness. And help relieve stress, and improve your physical and psychological well-being, by spending time outdoors, with Mother Nature!

" Everybody needs a place to play in. . .where nature may heal and cheer and give strength to body and soul alike. "
                                        -- John Muir, conservationist. 1915.

*****

The ability of the body to resist cancer and other diseases, viruses, sicknesses, and allergies depends on the condition of the immune system. We must have a strong and healthy immune system.

Because of environmental, ecological, and man-made influences (like convenience foods), our immune system cannot cope. Boost and restore the immune system with sufficient amino acids, essential fatty acids, vitamins, minerals, trace elements, and anti-oxidants.

Organically grown raw fruit especially, and to a lesser extent, raw vegetables, nuts and seeds contain all of these. They give energy and resistance, and build the immune system. Chemically produced fruit and vegetables are not nutritious or safe. We must demand organically grown produce and grains because no risks should be taken with something as vitally important as

71

our health. Anyway, it's no longer a risk, but an inevitability.

Many of today's health problems are self-induced, the result of the failure of the immune system. When under stress the immune system has to work extra hard, causing the body to produce less interferon, making the body's immune response deficient. Prevent disease by rebuilding the immune system.

We must take care of the body's defense system, which is the immune system. The most important rule is to follow as closely as possible the laws of Nature. Survival and fitness are reliant upon the ability to adapt to, and resist, the outside world.

The immune system is three types of cells: B-lymphocytes, T-lymphocytes, and macrophages. They work together, attacking bacteria, foreign invaders, and toxic substances like cancer and viruses. Bone marrow transplants save lives because bone marrow is the basis of your immune system. Emotional, mental, and physical disharmony causes problems with the immune system. Mind control and positive visualization and good actions are very important, therefore, for cure and prevention. Also, the immune system can be strengthened with evening primrose oil, borage oil, flax oil, or gammoleic acid. The immune system must be strong enough to withstand attacks from outside influences.

* * * * *

Nature provided for a healthy immune system to be maintained by eating raw fruit and vegetables, and seeds and nuts. Man-made food destroys the white blood cells and antibodies of the immune system, and inhibits the body's natural ability to make them.

Because of how and where we live, and have lived all our lives, our immune systems are deficient. Restore, rebuild, enhance your immune system for avoidance of diseases.

Social groups, cultures, groups of people that have little or no cancer, diabetes, heart disease, etc., obviously have strong and healthy immune systems. Always, these identified groups of people live in a chemically-free (at least relatively) environment; and always, organically grown fresh fruit, vegetables, and/or grain are major components of their diet -- often eaten raw.

Allergies are usually caused by a hypersensitive immune system. The immune system perceives innocent factors as invaders, and summons cellular defending forces to destroy it, or them. Balance must be restored to the immune system.

How? Detoxification is essential, as it is for cure and prevention of all diseases. But the faster the toxins are released and dissolved into the bloodstream, the greater the danger of overload. So a modified fast is necessary, first, then a change to natural foods.

Cancer, AIDS, and rheumatoid arthritis are immune system diseases. Remember that prescription drugs can destroy your immune system, and that vitamins A, C, E, selenium, beta carotene, and garlic enhance the immune system. Also, the immune system can be built up with ginseng, magnesium, EFA's, all B-vitamins, and all anti-oxidants.

"Orthodox doctors do not treat through diet
or strengthening the immune system. Thus,
the underlying disease remains dormant, and
will erupt and spread through the body again."
                                        --Dr. Edward Wagner.
                        * * * * *

73

CHAPTER VII
SAY GOODBYE TO YOUR HEALTH PROBLEMS

Solutions are often remarkably simple! If you have intestinal or digestive trouble, ulcers, rheumatism, or arthritis, try this method: Begin with the juice of one lemon and one tablespoon cold-pressed olive oil in the morning, before eating. Increase to at least the juice of three lemons and three tablespoons olive oil. Wait 15 minutes before eating. Also, drink as much lemon juice with water (and honey if you want) as you desire daily. Or try herbal teas. The herb shepherd's purse dissolves gallstones and the herb silymarin restores liver function. Peppermint oil tablets, used in Europe for many years, stop indigestion and ulcers. They are called Altoids at your drug or grocery store.

If you have heart disease you should eat fresh fruit and vegetables only. No alcohol, meat, white bread, milk, coffee, sugar, salt, or processed food. Herbal teas may help -- especially rosemary, thyme, and marigold. The heart must be detoxified. Also, try one teaspoon Montmorillonite clay with one-half glass water before breakfast. Also, lemon water, deep breathing, and sunshine. Any of these approaches will show results after weeks, not days. The condition took a long time to develop and cannot be remedied overnight. All holistic health approaches, in fact, may take at least five days to show change. Be patient, and you will be rewarded.

If you have liver problems use no dairy food. Cleanse the blood and liver with no solid food. Use one teaspoon clay with one-half cup water in the morning.

After any meal, take one-half lemon in one cup of hot water with honey.

In general, bed rest builds up the body's defenses. Therefore, it's a necessary part of any healing process.

* * * * *

Clay absorbs impurities, revitalizes the organs, stimulates glandular function. Use only fine quality clay, from health food stores. Results can be amazing when taken internally or used externally.

These are the foods to be eaten for good health: organic fresh fruits; sun dried fruits; cereals that are natural, unprocessed, and whole grain; whole grain wheat and rye breads that are sourdough, not yeast; fresh, organically grown vegetables; black olives; cold-pressed olive and flaxseed oils; sea salt; honey -- preferably rosemary; unprocessed fruit juice; herbal teas; filtered water or distilled water; sunflower seeds and nuts (unsalted); brown rice.

Foods to eat in moderation: two to four eggs weekly from chickens nourished naturally with grains and not raised in factories, as is commonly found in grocery stores; homemade pastry; legumes -- fresh peas and beans; fresh cheese and butter; sugarless jam.

* * * * *

The constitution of, and osmotic pressure of, sea water is similar to human blood. Therefore, always use sea salt, not common table salt which is detrimental to your health.

Foods to avoid are: all meat, animal fat, margarine, pasteurized butter, some fish because of water contamination, cooked oils (hydrogenated or polyunsaturated), canned or processed food, white flour, white rice, sugar, refined table salt, and pasteurized, homogenized milk.

Avoid foods that have been irradiated. Nuclear irradiation of foods produces mutations of chemicals with unforeseen consequences. Ask your grocer which of his food, which vegetables and fruit, are irradiated. Then tell him you will not buy it, and insist on organically grown produce. Money talks.

Meat brings toxic substances to the intestines and liver. It causes hardening of the blood vessels. Our society pressures us to eat meat. Not because it's good for us but because it's a huge industry. BIG BUSINESS. Meat is full of additives, hormones, drugs. Poisons. *Thousands* of studies have shown animal derived foods cause 75% of chronic diseases. And meat has to be cooked to be eaten. All these should be enough reasons not to eat meat, even if you're not bothered by the cruel, inhumane methods used to raise and kill animals that are eaten by you, and too many others.

Meat is not essential to human survival. You can get all the nutrients in meat from vegetable sources, except some B vitamins, which you can get from dairy products or brewer's yeast.

A very comprehensive book about food that is good for you, with recipes, is *The Whole Food Bible* by Christopher Kilham.

If you want to grow organic food on the least amount of land (200 to 300 square feet), with the least amount of water, working only 10 to 30 minutes a day then a book called *How to Grow More Vegetables (than you ever thought possible on less land than you can imagine)* by John Jeavons, will be very helpful.

Proper digestion, efficient assimilation, and regular elimination are requirements for good health. So, you are what you eat, digest, assimilate, and eliminate.

Food allergies are a common cause of indigestion. Insufficient enzymes are another. A deficiency of lactobacillus acidophilus is another. Fresh yogurt -- not commercially produced -- increases production of interferon and lactobacillus acidophilus. This can greatly improve health. It improves digestion, assimilation, and elimination. Lactobacillus acidophilus supplements will also help a lot.

Bromelain is a natural enzyme found in pineapple. This helps increase the body's ability to digest and break down fat from food. Cooking, food processing, canning, etc., eliminates live enzymes in our diet. This digestive enzyme can also have exceptional anti-inflammatory action. It reduces pain, inflammation, and swelling by reducing the harmful prostaglandins that cause pain and inflammation, and block the absorption of nutrients through the tissues. By helping to inhibit these pro-inflammatory substances, bromelain encourages well-nourished tissue that is free of pain and inflammation. It helps the healing process because it allows beneficial prostaglandins to work faster. It also maintains healthy joints, and may help allergies.

Aspirin inhibits *all* prostaglandins -- good and bad. Bromelain accomplishes the same thing as one aspirin a day does for your heart, only better. And it's natural.

Papaya provides more complete enzymes than bromelain, and therefore might be even more effective as a supplement. Take at least 200 mg. daily of either one, before meals.

Enzymes, in general, reinforce the immune system. Drugs, on the other hand, decrease the amount of antibodies in the body, which weakens the body's defenses -- the immune system. Drugs usually treat the symptoms, not the causes, and interfere with the body's natural immune system. Enzymes can be a safe alternative, because they stimulate the body's defenses. They catalyze normal body functions, and assist the immune system in detoxifying and eliminating wastes and toxins.

Enzymes are the foundation of life itself. They help everything in the body to function. This includes nerve impulses, regulation of hormones, cell renewal, production of energy, waste removal, and all metabolic processes, including immunological activities. In one minute one enzyme can be involved in 36 *million* biochemical reactions. This is more than amazing!

Enzymes made our planet able to be inhabited by allowing plants to produce oxygen. Enzymes are the most important biochemical in any living thing. Without enzymes there would be no life.

Enzymes are protein building blocks. They cause internal fermentation, which is the breakdown of organic compounds by the action of enzymes. They work synergistically with vitamins, minerals, and trace elements. Vitamins and minerals are co-enzymes, meaning they combine with enzymes to function. They are involved in the reactions of enzymes.

Health, which is harmony and balance of all biological processes, depends on enzymes. Illness, or disharmony and imbalance, results from enzyme imbalance. Deficiencies can result in problems as simple as fatigue, headaches, digestive problems, or memory loss. Or, problems as complicated as cancer, old age, and chronic disease. Wounds heal faster and better with external application of enzymes.

Supplementation with enzymes could revolutionize medicine. In Europe, 500 million tablets of Wobenzymes (a highly purified enzyme formula/combination) are sold each year. Bromelain, papaya, and pancreatic enzymes are the most easily attainable, in the United States, from health food sources. Or, raw, fresh, organic vegetables and fruits also supply enzymes.

* * * * *

Diet related diseases cause about 300,000 deaths a year, according to the American Medical Association. Former U.S. Surgeon General Dr. C. Everett Koop attributes about 75% of all degenerative diseases in the U.S. to diet. And, according to the Journal of the American Medical Association, alcoholism is the cause of death for about 100,000 people a year.

Independent studies have revealed that individuals who improve their nutrition while in the Alcoholics Anonymous 12 Step Program have a far greater chance of success. Recovery from addictions to food, alcohol, and drugs will be much more successful when proper nutrition is followed, and chemicals are eliminated from our food. Nutritional treatment influences repair of the body at the cellular level.

Degenerative diseases originate from enzyme deficiencies. The body's inability to fight cancer is a result of inadequate nutrition and the inability of the pancreas to produce enzymes. *The food ingested must be absorbed.*

Supplement a diet with digestive enzymes, which break down food elements to be absorbed for optimal nutrition and energy. Cooking above 118° F kills all enzymes. Treatment with enzymes and supplementary vitamins and minerals have yielded remarkable results. Enzyme therapy alone has no side effects and often gives miraculous results. It is especially invaluable in incurable degenerative diseases. Additionally, most degenerative diseases have a manganese deficiency.

Instead of killing cells (with drugs), it is better to assist healthy cells to fight abnormal cells. As an example, in the case of cancer it is a fight between the regenerative cells and the degenerative cells.

Germanium is an outstanding immune enhancer. It inhibits cell multiplication, stops damage created by radiation and radioactivity, increases production of interferon, increases absorption of calcium, lessens pain, gives energy, improves heart muscle tone, and removes mercury and other metal poisons from the body. It also enriches the body's oxygen supply. (Because of increased carbon dioxide in the air, all human oxygen absorption is under threat. Since plants and trees turn carbon dioxide into oxygen, it is obvious we also need more plants and trees.) It destroys toxic free-radicals, and discharges poisons from the system.

Ginseng has germanium in it, as does aloe, comfrey, and garlic. Ginseng has been in continual daily use by millions for more than 5,000 years. Yet, Western society (i.e. the medical establishment) thinks it needs to be "scientifically" tested and validated. It is used to restore homeostasis -- the body's balance -- or to normalize various body functions like blood pressure, blood sugar, hormones, and energy. Health and vitality, energy, and a positive attitude are benefits of taking ginseng. Also, it helps asthma, fatigue, stress, diabetes, impotence, metabolism, and builds the immune system. It may help tumors and cancer.

The water of Lourdes, France -- famous for its healing properties -- has germanium in it. This mineral has been used in other countries with remarkable results. It acts as a catalyzer, enhancing the creation of white and red blood cells, and also dissolves abnormal cells. A noted physician said giving oxygen to the cells is the ideal way to cure diseases. Organic germanium does this immediately.

Garlic is a natural detoxifier and potent immune stimulant. It has germanium and selenium in it. It protects from damage due to chemicals, heavy metals, radiation, and stress. Garlic and yogurt are the best for reducing cholesterol. People who eat garlic regularly are 1000 times less likely to suffer from stomach and pancreatic cancers! Garlic and olive oil are components of one of the best diets in the world -- the Mediterranean diet. It is found in capsules at grocery stores and health food stores. It destroys viruses, lowers blood pressure, and is a proven antibiotic owing to its high sulphur content. To eliminate excess candidas albicans use garlic and olive oil. Garlic helps indigestion, bronchitis, arthritis and rheumatism.

Aloe vera has been known to cause remarkable healing. Because of individual body chemistry and severity of problems, healing time can vary a lot. Sometimes it takes longer than 60 days to see and feel beneficial results. It is a natural anti-inflammatory and detoxifying agent that stimulates your body's own repair system. Healing time is therefore relative to the problem. (This is, of course, true with all natural healing methods.) Cold-pressed pure aloe vera, taken full strength, stimulates and increases the body's natural ability to heal

81

itself. For centuries, it has been widely used for arthritis, colitis, diverticulitis, ulcers, dry skin, itching, gum problems, indigestion, constipation, hemorrhoids, hair loss, and to heal wounds, breaks, burns, inflammation, and diaper rash.

Health From God's Garden, by Maria Treben from Austria, has very effective remedies for many health problems. To prevent or restore hair loss use burdock, walnut, or nettle herb rinses. If you're tired and listless, or have gallstones, eat dandelion stems, 10 a day for two weeks; chew well. (Wash with flowers still on to retain juice.) For a blood purifier and inner cleanser drink nettle, yarrow, and dandelion teas. For kidney stones use nettle tea. For nerves, paralysis, sinus, insomnia, infections use St. John's wort, chamomile, thyme, sage teas, and Swedish bitters.

* * * * *

After 30 years of practice as a cardiologist, Dr. Bruno Cortis wrote in his book, *Heart and Soul,* that "People have the power to heal themselves if they will assume personal responsibility for their health."

Most of the diseases and sicknesses we suffer are self-inflicted, or society-inflicted. You can often cure yourself through better nutrition because the body can then repair itself.

Nutritional therapy supports the defensive mechanisms. It often gets rid of the biochemical cause of problems, not just the symptoms. Sickness results from inefficient use of oxygen. Efficient use of oxygen enables the body to defend itself successfully against infecting organisms. Proper nutrition increases the body's defenses which are dependent upon efficient use of oxygen.

82

Therapeutic nutrition is perhaps the medicine of the near future, as Thomas Edison predicted many years ago.

*****

Nutritional medicine reestablishes homeostasis. It never controls the disease or sickness, as chemical drugs attempt to do. That is why nutritional approaches take longer to see results.

The solution to living in peace and harmony and health is to create balance. The state of health is balance. Nutritional imbalances cause health problems. Behavior problems and physiological problems can be directly connected with what we eat and drink.

Such simple solutions as high potency brewer's yeast and high potency vitamin C often help restore balance in chronic health problems. Grapeseed extract may eliminate ADD (Attention Deficit Disorder).

U.S. Secretary of Health and Human Services, Louis Sullivan, said in 1990: "We can no longer ignore the fact that prevention is the most important factor in maintaining good health." The key to prevention is lifestyle, a different approach to living. Not early detection of problems, but prevention of problems.

*****

Being overweight is one of the most common results of inefficient nutrition. Extra weight is a symptom of inefficiencies in the conversion and elimination process. Specifically -- conversion of food into energy and tissue and waste, and elimination of that waste.

As an example, as we get older our ability to use chromium decreases. About 90% of Americans have a chromium deficiency. This trace element influences fat and cholesterol metabolism, calorie burning, hunger control, and enhancement of the action of insulin. It increases longevity, and increases muscle mass. A naturally occurring form is found in plant tissue. Another example is that a deficiency of EFA's causes blood sugar levels to fall, and causes a person to feel hungry all the time. Weight gain is inevitable.

Losing weight can be a matter of increasing efficiency of digestion and elimination. Enzymes or lactobacillus acidophilus taken before you eat, or fresh fruit (containing enzymes) eaten before you eat other food (like the ancient Romans did), will help digestion. Better digestion = more energy = weight loss and general well-being. Also, take chromium supplements and EFA's. More fiber, or psyllium powder (Metamucil® or generic), increases elimination. An inner cleansing product like Arise and Shine might cause you to lose ten pounds the first week you use it.

High calorie malnutrition. This sounds wrong, and is worse than wrong. It is modern day, affluent starvation. Empty calories, empty food, artificial food, and chemical nutrition. Empty calories do not satisfy your body's need for nutrition. You feel hungry so you eat more. An inability to digest food means less nutrients being assimilated. Digestion is what provides our bodies with fuel, with energy, with restorative capabilities. Inadequate digestion means problems somewhere, sometime.

Environmental stresses cause inefficient digestion, metabolism, immune systems, and insufficient energy and recovery. They also cause toxicity, hormone

84

imbalances, and emotional stresses. Nutrition and herbal support help neutralize these negative effects.

The body has its own natural repair mechanisms that need to be encouraged, supported, improved. Drugs suppress these repair capabilities, treating symptoms not causes. Traditional doctors treat symptoms, not causes, and as such they cause *more* problems.

James Frackelton, M.D., past president of the American College for Advancement in Medicine said: "Traditional orthodox medicine has taken on all the characteristics of a religion, and any threat to its *status quo* is unfortunately treated as heresy. Our present course will bankrupt our country without having the desired results of good, effective medicine. "

The better way is nutritional medicine, because it influences repair at the cellular level. Also, adequate sleep, pure water, adequate oxygen, appropriate exercise, adequate digestion and elimination of wastes, and eliminating or neutralizing environmental stresses.

Dr.Linus Pauling said:

" I believe that you can, by taking some simple and inexpensive measures, lead a longer and healthier life. The most important recommendation is that you take vitamins everyday in optimum amounts, much larger than that recommended by physicians and old-fashioned nutritionists. "

* * * * *

Dr.Bernard Jensen said, "It is the intestinal system that has to be cared for, first, before any effective healing

85

can take place." Many people agree that detoxification of the body is the key to health and youth. Usually, the amount of toxicity directly correlates with the severity of the health problem. These include fatigue, weight gain, arthritis, cancer, body odor, constipation, bloating, skin problems, etc.

In the 1970's, L. Ron Hubbard (Church of Scientology) developed a detoxification technique called the Purification Program for drug/chemical accumulation and contamination, which leads to chemically related disease and health problems. (His book: *Clear Body, Clear Mind*.) It utilizes saunas, oils, niacin, vitamins, minerals, water, potassium, and exercise. His purpose was to help people get rid of toxins, which are deposited mainly in fat tissue, thereby slowing mental and spiritual advancement.

A poorly functioning eliminative system results in toxic accumulation. This leads to development of degenerative diseases, or health disorders. Built up toxins in the colon are absorbed into the bloodstream. Health and vitality are diminished. Internal cleansing (detoxification) may alleviate or help *any* health complaint.

After inner cleansing, it is imperative to have proper nutrition to avoid a repetition of the problem(s). You really are what you eat!

Seventy-five percent of the human body is water. It flushes toxins, wastes, and cellular debris from our body, and transports nutrients for assimilation. That's why drinking 8 glasses a day is necessary.

Twenty to thirty minutes a day of heart rate elevation causes the lymphatic system to circulate and cleanse the body. Without exercise the lymphatic fluid can't circulate.

A juice fast of at least three days removes stress from organs and digestive processes, allowing healing and rebuilding.

Poor eating habits lead to problems in the intestinal tract which later may develop into chronic and degenerative diseases. About 90% of health problems can be caused by an unhealthy digestive system. One reason for this is a gradual buildup of many layers of mucoid placque substance in the intestinal tract.

We need to get rid of the reason for the problem, to deal with causes, not symptoms. Sir Jason Winters overcame cancer with his herbal combinations, which he later marketed worldwide. He said, "If a person purifies the blood of toxins and environmental pollutants, oxygen and nutrition can travel to every part of the body. Nourish and purify your body and I believe that poor health goes scurrying." Dr. Bernard Jensen says, "Internal cleansing is the key to youth, vitality, energy, and vibrant health."

Arise & Shine Herbal Products in Tucson, Arizona has a "clean-me-out" program based on herbs. For more information call 1-800-688-2444.

Homozon is an herbal product for these purposes from Aerobic Life in Pheonix, Arizona (1-800-798-0707). Also, superior healing power is found in the herb hyssop, which means "holy herb". Since the beginning of time it has been used to cleanse and purify the body.

* * * * *

It is possible to partially detoxify your body by using herbal teas and capsules without any kind of fasting, thereby not interfering with daily routine or the common preoccupation with food and eating. These eliminate toxins from the organs that filter toxins -- the liver, the kidneys, and intestines. Constipation, bloating, improper digestion, loss of energy, and chronic fatigue should be stopped after about two weeks of this type of cleansing. Detoxification from chemicals or metals is possible with ginkgo biloba, niacin, CoQ10, and brewer's yeast.

The Health Center for Better Living at 6189 Taylor Road, Naples, Florida 33942 will send "A Useful Guide to Herbal Health Care" free, if you request one. They have a comprehensive line of herbal products. Their motto is: "God has given us herbs as food for our better health and better living. "

Dandelion tea, chamomile tea, and alfalfa tea can help detoxify poisons in the liver, and lower blood pressure. Dandelion also breaks up fatty deposits in veins and arteries. Comfrey tea or capsules fight infections, and kidney and bladder ailments. It also helps heal burns and cuts. Dong quai herbs maintain proper hormone balance for women, and help menstrual disorders. Eyebright is good for weak eyesight. Gentian root helps the liver and digestive organs.

There are hundreds of herbs to investigate, if you are interested. Many herbs have medicinal values, and all should be used with caution, and never taken in excessive quantities. Also, always take with a glass of water, or as tea. Start with a small amount of herbs, and increase gradually, as seems appropriate.

Chinese doctors have used kudzu for gastrointestinal problems and alcoholism for more than a thousand years. Valerian root has been used for sleep disorders, headaches, nervousness, exhaustion, and anxiety for thousands of years. Hence the drug Valium.

Approximately 80% of the U.S. pharmacopoeia was originally derived from herb and plant substances.

A free catalog of herbs is available from Brion Herbs, a distributor of herbs since 1948. Their number is 1-800-777-2309. Also, Indiana Botanic Gardens, established 1910, has a very interesting catalog (free) at 1-800-644-TEAS. Transpacific Health products at 1-800-336-9636 also has a free catalog of Chinese teas.

* * * * *

Carpal tunnel syndrome is associated with numbness, tingling, or shooting pains. It is confirmed with a simple test devised by Dr. John Ellis in his book *Vitamin B6: The Doctor's Report*. This test is done by touching the fingertips to the palm of the hand at the base of each finger, all at the same time. If unable to do this, an advanced deficiency of vitamin B6, or pyridoxine, is very probable. The solution to this problem is 50 to 200 mg. of B6, three times a day, with high potency B-complex, also three times a day (at the same time). The high potency, which is harmless, is necessary to "get out of the hole" created by years of vitamin B6 and B-complex deficiency. To this, add 200 mg. magnesium citrate, and one tablespoon EFA's (cold-pressed soy, sunflower, safflower, etc., oils) -- both twice a day. These are B6 co-factors. (If one nutrient is deficient, the others probably are too.) Taking these B vitamins will also lower your risk of strokes and heart attacks.

* * * * *

89

Chronic fatigue is a common complaint. Stress, depression, chronic fatigue, and lack of energy may be alleviated with the use of high potency brewer's yeast, or Ultimate Green, which combines chlorella, algae, wheat and barley grass, spinach, alfalfa, and herbal enzymes.

Chronic fatigue begins in the digestive tract (faulty digestion and malabsorption of essential nutrients) and ends with toxic by-products being reabsorbed into the body. The digestive process is the key factor in maintaining optimum health and adequate energy. Nutrients have to be absorbed and assimilated. Undigested food can ferment in the 98.6° F digestive tract and become toxic, eventually polluting all tissues and cells. Food allergies and chronic fatigue can result.

An internal cleansing program is the first step. Herb and fiber combinations, and fresh juice, should do this. Organic whole grains, fruit, and vegetables (no processed food) help alleviate chronic fatigue and keep it from returning. Converting that food into nutrients for energy may require enzyme supplementation. B-complex vitamins (brewer's yeast is best) also raise energy levels, sometimes as much as 90%. Therapeutic supplementation can change people's lives by strengthening their immune system and improving their lives in general. This also includes the so-called green superfoods: chlorella, spirulina, blue-green algae, wheat and barley grass, and spinach, all of which are extremely nutrient dense and easily assimilated. Assimilating optimum nourishment provides optimum health, and will eliminate chronic fatigue.

* * * * *

Fluoride increases the rate of cancer by 26%. Chlorine kills parasites and bacteria in water. It also poisons you and causes heart disease. The purest water to drink is distilled water.

Drugs, including aspirin and birth control pills, are toxic to the thyroid gland. So is chlorine and fluoride. Thyroid deficiency is a major cause of heart disease. People with heart disease usually are deficient in thyroid hormone, magnesium, and CoQ10. Thyroid problems indicate a need for vitamin A, CoQ10, zinc, magnesium, and minerals. As we age thyroid problems and zinc deficiencies become more common. A dry, furry sensation in the mouth may indicate a zinc deficiency. However, it may take months of 30 to 50 mg. of elemental zinc each day to improve a thyroid problem.

The thyroid is responsible for our basal metabolic rate (metabolism), which is the rate the body burns calories for energy. Hypothyroidism is an underactive thyroid, a sluggish metabolism resulting in fatigue, weight gain and feeling cold and/or depressed. This condition impairs the function of every organ, tissue, and cell. It becomes impossible to break down food properly, and assimilate nutrients. Kelp is a natural source of iodine, necessary for normal thyroid function. Also, vitamin C (500 mg. to 1000 mg. a day) is beneficial to thyroid functioning.

Moodiness, anxiety, and inferiority complexes can be related to iodine deficiencies affecting the thyroid. Fresh green vegetables and minerals are helpful in maintaining emotional stability determined by the thyroid.

* * * * *

Heart bypass surgery is a traumatic, high risk procedure. It has been estimated 87,500 people have this done needlessly each year. About 350,000 bypass surgeries are performed yearly. So, about 25% of the total are done unnecessarily. In some hospitals, one out of every five patients dies. Other risks are strokes and heart attacks. Also, some brain injury is very likely because of the heart-lung machine used during the operation.

Statistics show that 50% of all bypass grafts are clogged again within five years, and 80% within seven years. Bypass operations have been shown over and over again to have no effect on women's life expectancy. About 300,000 balloon angioplasties are done yearly, and no study has shown them to be more effective than non-surgical approaches. How many people are aware of these frightening odds before they go through this ordeal?

The cost per patient is about $25,000 to $40,000. This brings in about $10 *billion* dollars a year to the medical community. This is BIG BUSINESS.

EDTA chelation therapy is a safe, effective, and low-cost alternative to open heart surgery. It is a painless, non-surgical method for opening up clogged arteries that is used around the world -- except in the USA. It targets the main arteries leading to your heart and the entire 75,000 miles of blood vessels in the circulatory system. For a list of physicians offering chelation therapy call: 1-800-LEAD OUT. EDTA chelation therapy dissolves placque inside the arteries to increase blood flow. The improved circulation happens gradually. This safe, painless, and 100% legal procedure needs to be available for everyone. Why isn't it? The answer is obvious.

The Chelation Way by Dr. Morton Walker is recommended.

* * * * *

Candidiasis was described by Hippocrates in 400 B.C. However, not until recently has it been diagnosed as the reason for a multitude of problems. An overgrowth of yeast causes chronic fatigue, herpes simplex, viruses, parasites, constipation, diarrhea, bloating, acne, rashes, blurred vision and other eye problems, infection or fluid in ears, nasal congestion, gum/mouth/throat problems, urinary and vaginal problems, weight problems, irritability, headaches, and food allergies.

The causes for the candidiasis, or overgrowth of yeast, are a weakened immune system, repeated use of antibiotics, excess sugar and carbohydrates, birth control pills, and EFA (essential fatty acid) deficiency.

We normally have over 300 types of yeast and fungi on our skin alone. Hundreds more are in the gastrointestinal and genital areas. When they proliferate abnormally they change to a fungus and cause a diversity of problems.

Yeast infections are more common than you might think. In fact, they affect about 75 million people. It has been called the disease of the century, because of the common use of antibiotics for about 50 years, and because of the presence of antibiotics in animal flesh eaten commonly by the population. Yeast infections are caused by candida albicans. Antibiotics wipe out good bacteria in the intestines and yeast then takes over, gets out of control, and poisons the whole body. It can then be one of the causes of arthritis, autism, asthma, psoriasis, infertility, insomnia, PMS, indigestion, depression, and a depressed immune system. Una de gato, D-yeast, pau d'arco, Immunex, and other specifically combined herbs to eliminate yeast infections are available from health food stores. Lactobacillus acidophilus tablets/capsules are a good preventative and healing measure, restoring beneficial bacteria in the intestines.

Another common health problem is arthritis. More Americans, (at least 30 million people), suffer from arthritis than any other chronic ailment. If you suffer with arthritis, a change in diet may cure or relieve it. It may be caused by food allergies. Avoid red meat, white flour, white sugar, refined salt, and possibly tomatoes and potatoes. Increase intake of fresh, uncooked fruit and vegetables, whole grain food, and distilled water. Avoid sodium nitrates and preservatives. Exercise (daily walks, etc.) every day. Avoid stress and constipation. A natural source of cortisone for arthritis are yucca plant tablets. Also, aloe vera, Co-enzyme Q10, and Willard Water will help. Vitalife products (1-800-749-3937) has Arthritis Ease –very helpful for arthritis. Juice fasts can be very beneficial also. Glucosamine is a natural compound found in high concentrations in joint spaces. It stimulates production of connective tissue and repair of joints that are arthritic.

* * * * *

Cancer cannot exist in a balanced metabolic system. So, when balance is restored, malignancy will often slow down or regress. Conventional medical approaches for cancer and tumors seek and destroy – or try to destroy. Maybe destroying the good, the bad, the ugly. And the beautiful. Maybe not.

Cancer and multiple sclerosis are immune deficiency syndromes. Vitamins A, C, D, E, all other anti-oxidants, garlic, the minerals zinc, iron, manganese, and selenium, all promote a healthy immune system.

94

For cancer and leukemia chelated mineral supplementation is necessary. These minerals include calcium, iron, selenium, iodine, phosphorus, zinc, potassium, chromium, magnesium, and copper. The digestive system of the cancer patient is severely overtaxed. Enzyme supplementation is necessary.

Cancer steals nutrients from normal tissue and blood, necessitating extra vitamins, minerals, and enzymes, as would any sickness. The sick body does not have enough enzymes to digest food, and to digest and assimilate protein. A natural and healthy diet strengthens the immune system, thereby increasing chances of survival with cancer and leukemia.

One out of three people now falls victim to some form of cancer. Many years ago, it was determined that proteolytic enzymes are responsible for the destruction of malignant cells. Why was this extremely important discovery ignored? Why wasn't it incorporated into cancer treatment long ago? Why not now? Wobe-mucos or Wobenzyme tablets from Germany contain several kinds of proteolytic enzymes which have proven to be highly successful. Why aren't they used in the U. S.? Guess. Years ago, the American scientist Richard Will Statler was asked when a cure for cancer would be discovered. He said, "When cancer is cured, it will be by enzyme action." However, there will be no cure for cancer until the medical establishment – a giant industry – allows it.

If all the genes in a cell operate simultaneously then disorganized growth occurs, and the name for that is cancer. It is possible to stop cancer growth and live comfortably for many years, but still have cancer. It is possible to control it and live a fulfilling life. People who follow an appropriate diet, and refrain from excesses or indulgences, can control cancer and leukemia. This has been proven repeatedly. A macrobiotic diet is especially beneficial.

Viruses can be a contributing factor to cancer. The body's healthy cells must be helped in their fight against any abnormal cells. Viruses must be treated properly in their early stages. Also, if the body's system cannot remove artificial additives, colors, preservatives, fertilizers, etc., which invade healthy cells, then cancer cells can take over and healthy cells cannot form.

Holistic treatment for all health problems has a basic premise of no damage to normal cells. Non-toxic cancer treatment involves increased oxygenation, enzymes, vitamins, herbs, minerals, dietary management, and raw organic fruits and vegetables.

It is very important to visualize yourself as recovering. Often. And do deep breathing exercises daily for about fifteen minutes, to increase oxygen supplied to cells. Visualize the cancer cells being destroyed by the white cells many times a day. Visualize being well. Often. Repeat: "I will be victorious over my problems." Do this many times a day, to program the mind, like a computer, with a positive attitude. You can prevent and control, or overcome, many problems with this control of your mind. Psychoneuroimmunology theorizes that emotions and attitudes are connected with our nervous, endocrine, and immune systems.

Pau d'arco is made from the inner bark of the lapacho tree that grows in southern Brazil. As tea or tablets/capsules it relieves pain, cures some diabetes, arthritis, and some cancer. It eliminates toxins, purifies the blood, and is anti-fungal. Chronic yeast infections can be cleared up. It is anti-inflammatory, and increases red blood cells. I know from experience that it can eliminate tumors, and help leukemia and other health problems.

Beres Drops, a Hungarian remedy rich in certain trace elements and minerals, helps cancer patients, emphasizing quality -- not quantity.

Shark cartilage reputedly changes tumors to a jelly-like substance, thereby eliminating some forms of cancer. It may also be helpful for arthritis. Bovine cartilage reportedly is even more effective.

A woman in Brea, California who used "Staff of Life" products said, "In 1991, my father had leukemia and was failing fast. After taking L.Salivarias, amylase, and protease enzymes for about three months, his doctor announced, "No more leukemia! A miracle! "

Vitamin B17 is laetrile. It is found in apricot kernels and raw almonds. Why is the medical establishment against this repeatedly proven cancer remedy? Perhaps vitamin B17 therapy is too easy an answer, with little profit potential. However, careful handling, monitoring, and administration are essential.

Essiac tea, originally from Canadian Indians, has helped many thousands of people eliminate, lessen, or put in remission, many kinds of cancer. It also improves health in general.

*****

When the viscosity of the blood is good and circulation is good, the growth of the secondary cancer will be limited. It is unusual to perish from primary tumors. A spontaneous remission is possible with a diet including high potency vitamins, minerals, trace elements, enzymes, and either germanium, B17, una de gato, Essiac, or pau d'arco. Recovery is only possible when the immune system can be regenerated, when liver function is stimulated, and the patient has a positive attitude.

To prevent cancer have a good oxygen supply; prevent constipation; have good blood circulation and chemistry; avoid overweight; exclude fats, animal protein, toxic material, nicotine, and alcohol; avoid aluminum cooking utensils; use extra vitamins, minerals, and trace elements; avoid drugs if possible; get plenty of exercise in fresh air; use sea salt (Celtic) in moderation instead of table salt. And remember that the endocrine system is very sensitive to thoughts, emotions, and actions, and visual experiences. Positive visualization is important for both cure and prevention. And don't forget enzyme supplementation.

Repeatedly, it has been proven that leukemia can be a result of nuclear fallout, from nuclear reactors. High dosages of vitamin C, kelp, and calcium-magnesium-zinc can be of great help. Symptoms of acute leukemia are almost identical to those of scurvy. Therefore, vitamin C is essential in its treatment and prevention.

To aid the production of new cells in chemotherapy treatment (not recommended) use extra vitamins, minerals, and trace elements.

Cancer Blackout, a book by Nat Morris, reveals a 200 year history of the development, use, and suppression of many successful, non-toxic cancer remedies.

Another useful book is *Options for Alternative Cancer Therapy*, by Richard Walters. Maureen Salaman says that cancer deaths can be prevented by using the information in her book, *Nutrition – The Cancer Answer*.

A concentrated fermented soybean extract called Haelan 851, from China, allows cells to help themselves and, thereby, has helped cure cancer and Alzheimer's (1-800-542-3526).

Wobenzyme tablets are pancreatin, trypsin, chymotrypsin, bromelain, papain, and rutosid. For a free sample of Wobenzymes write the exclusive United States distributor: Naturally Vitamins, 14851 North Scottsdale Road, Scottsdale, Arizona 85254.

*****

Recent studies have shown that a shortage of progesterone, not estrogen, causes heart attacks and other problems in post-menopausal women. Almost as many women have heart attacks as men. Yes, it's true.

Estrogen used in Premarin pills is horse urine. (Pre=prenatal, mar=mare, in=urine.) Pregnant female horses are confined in a small stall during the first six months of their pregnancy. They cannot lay down, but must *stand* for the entire six months with a bag to catch urine attached to them. After this hideously cruel procedure they are often arthritic or crippled. Their baby colts, born about five months later, are usually destroyed or sent to the slaughterhouse. If you want to risk using estrogen pills (cancer, etc.) consider using synthetic. Better yet, use natural estrogen.

Menopause is a simple hormonal change in the reproductive status of women. The hormonal system needs to be balanced so the body can adjust to its new status, and to avoid any discomforts. Natural sources of estrogen are black cohosh and red raspberry herbs, dates, raisins, grapes, apples, peaches, almonds, and peanuts. Both progesterone and estrogen are found in wild yam and sarsparilla herbs. Ginseng has phytoestrogens which help hormonal balance. Una de gato and suma also balance hormones. Vitamins C, B6, and B12 may help. Enzymes are needed for every chemical action and reaction in the body. This includes hormone function. Boron supplements, or naturally occurring boron, may increase mental alertness, calcium assimilation, and estrogen levels as much as estrogen replacement therapy. Dates, apples, and peaches are good sources of boron. If they are not cooked they also provide enzymes.

The chaste tree berry, suma, and dong quai restore monthly regularity, and may relieve symptoms of menopause. In both cases it is necessary to restore estrogen-progesterone balance.

Increased cholesterol levels are a natural occurrence with natural menopause, and induced (hysterectomy) menopause. Millions of women have been prescribed cholesterol lowering drugs. Studies show these drugs have unpleasant side effects in women, and do *not* increase life expectancy. Garlic, as an example, lowers cholesterol naturally.

In the past 50 years breast cancer has risen 86%. Before the year 2000 about two million women will be diagnosed with breast cancer, and about 500,000 will die. Approximately one woman every 12 minutes. Mammograms miss 10% to 15% of breast cancer and probably increase the risk of getting it. Remember, mammograms are early detection, not prevention. Any woman reading this will agree that prevention is necessary, that mammograms are not the answer to this deplorable and frightening problem.

More women are dying from heart attacks (about 360,000 each year) than ever before. How many women develop heart problems, or thyroid problems, after taking birth control pills for 5 to 25 years? Birth control pills are toxic to the thyroid gland. Thyroid deficiency is a major cause of heart disease. The connection seems to be clear.

* * * * *

Non-specific medical problems, ones unable to be given names or identified, are often due to severe stress, including environmental stresses. Problems that are supposedly psychological or psychosomatic may instead be nutritional imbalances. What is the person eating and drinking? Are there any prescription or non-prescription drugs being used? What about their lifestyle? Health is a state of equilibrium.

Inadequate levels of thiamine in babies three to four months old seems to be a cause of Sudden Infant Death Syndrome (SIDS). That risk can be eliminated with 10 to 50 mg. of thiamine, three times a day. Too much causes rapid heartbeat, so individual monitoring is necessary (by a physician). This was discovered by Dr.Derrick Lonsdale, M.D., who says in his book *Why I Left Orthodox Medicine*: "Nutritional medicine will be the mandatory medicine of the next century. . . It is extremely effective."

More than 50 medical problems are caused or provoked by allergic reactions to food. These include arthritis, asthma, fatigue, headaches, weight gain or loss, and indigestion. (Asthma beginning after age 45 is usually due to infections.)

101

Hypoglycemia is called the underdiagnosed problem. A lot of sugar or carbohydrates at one time make the level of blood sugar rise too high. It can be avoided by reducing the amount of insulin released while eating. Many small meals a day accomplishes this, instead of three. Regulate blood sugar levels, or relieve the symptoms of hypoglycemia, with chromium, ginseng, una de gato, EFA's, and pau d'arco. Hypoglycemia happens because of low blood chromium level, or low thyroid level. Therefore, kelp should also help.

Nearly a million people each year die from cardiovascular disease. More than one in five Americans are living now with some form of that disease. About 46% of all deaths in America can be attributed to cardiovascular disease. Magnesium and vitamin E can help.

Magnesium is one of the most important minerals for health. It is a catalyst to over 300 enzymatic reactions. Deficiency increases heart attack or stroke risk by *100 %*. If one is taking it at the time these occur then recovery is 83% more likely. (Take 300 mg. daily). Magnesium has a calming effect on the nervous system. Elevated pulse rates and heart arrhythmias can be due to a magnesium deficiency. Deficiency causes kidney stones, as does a high fat diet. About one person in ten will have kidney stones. Deficiency also intensifies thyroid problems, causes glaucoma, and Parkinson's disease tremors. Magnesium oxide is poorly absorbed, so use magnesium potassium aspartate or orotate. Vitamin E (400 I.U.) prevents blood clots. Magnesium and vitamin E taken daily will *prevent* most heart attacks and strokes. This is really amazing! It also helps diabetes, arthritis, lupus, and infertility. (Vitamin C has been used to increase

102

fertility in men.) Use only natural, non-esterfied vitamin E. Applied topically it can eliminate cysts.

Potassium deficiencies can cause heart pain and arrhythmias.

Co-enzyme Q10 increases muscle strength 56% (so it would be helpful for those in physical therapy), reduces risk of cancer, strengthens the heart and liver, reduces risk of heart attack, helps arthritis, delays aging, reduces cholesterol levels and high blood pressure, and improves the immune system. It has benefited cats with leukemia.

The saw palmetto tree provides a solution to maintaining male prostate health. The saw palmetto berry contains natural substances that are highly effective and beneficial in normalizing male hormones. It has been researched extensively in Europe. Why take Proscar? Also, zinc plays a major role in maintaining the function of the prostate. A Swedish study in 1992 found that of 223 men who were not treated for early prostate cancer, only 19 died from the disease within 10 years of diagnosis. Flaxseed oil (1000 to 1500 mg) helps about 70% of men with this problem. Testosterone levels are related to hair growth and loss.

An extract of Mexican yams is a naturally occurring form of estrogen, with no side effects like cancer or heart problems.

People with nervous disorders may have a shortage of calcium, manganese, and niacin. Niacin is also necessary for production of hydrochloric acid for digestion. It helps joint mobility (100 mg.).

Colloidal silver was used medically until the late 1930's, when it was replaced by antibiotics, primarily sulfa. It is a broad spectrum germicide, disabling the enzyme used by bacteria, viruses, and fungus. It is non-toxic.

An antibiotic kills about six different disease organisms, but silver kills about 650. Also, resistant strains fail to develop. So why aren't doctors using it? It's obvious why doctors aren't using it.

Superoxide dismatuse, an antioxidant, has been used by Princess Diana's step mother and thousands of others in Europe to prevent aging. It revitalizes the cells and reduces the rate of cell destruction. It also removes the most common free-radical, superoxide. For some people, it improves arthritis and joint problems.

Bananas are rich in potassium, lowering high blood pressure by as much as 40%.

Calcium helps prevent colon cancer. It is most effective taken as several small doses throughout the day. A continuous supply of calcium in the bloodstream is necessary to promote passage of nutrients through cell walls, for function of muscles, and to prevent removal of calcium from bone, which eventually causes osteoporosis (porous and brittle bones). Bones lose and gain calcium each day of your life, as they are constantly reformed. Calcium works synergistically with many other nutrients so it is best to take supplements with meals. Also, the acid produced from eating breaks down calcium. It is often difficult to assimilate calcium unless chelated or citrate.

Evening primrose oil has the essential fatty acids gamma linolenic and linoleic, derived from the flower's seeds. Black currant seed oil has these acids, also. They can help arthritis, multiple sclerosis, allergies, skin problems, menopause symptoms, inflammation, and muscular dystrophy.

Disease is often not the result of an enemy invader, but the absence of a necessary factor. An imbalance. As an example, anemia can lead to further health problems like infections. If you are anemic you are not getting enough oxygen to your cells, and a shortage of oxygen can lead to health problems involving bacteria, fungi, and viruses. Insufficient oxygen and anemia can cause fatigue, low energy, and poor resistance. Children who crave paint and mud are probably anemic. For cells to function at maximum capability they must have adequate oxygen. Mental acuity and better health are the result. This points to the value of exercise and adequate iron, since both increase oxygen, and to one of the dangers of air pollution. It takes 2-6 months for tissue to return to normal during treatment.

Free-radicals are a part of normal metabolism and are controlled if proper nutrients are available. Once free-radical activity is controlled natural healing processes can take over. *Free-radical damage is reversible with proper nutrition.* Beta carotene, vitamin E and C, selenium, niacin, and riboflavin are free-radical scavengers. Radiation produces free-radicals, but the greater dangers are free-radicals in our diet, and those produced by pollution. Premature aging and degenerative diseases result.

The most dangerous source of free-radicals are all unsaturated hydrogenated fats and rancid fats. (Use saturated fats for cooking because they don't oxidize, and *never* reuse heated oil. It's carcinogenic.) Other sources of free-radicals are natural and man-made radiation, the ozone, alcohol, tobacco smoke, chlorinated water, iron and copper excesses, and too little oxygen (from lack of exercise, etc.).

Free-radicals are molecules or atoms that are highly reactive. They are both essential to life processes and highly destructive. They detoxify and give energy, and kill invading bacteria. But when out of control they are very destructive, producing cellular damage leading to cancer, aging, etc.

The synergistic effects of vitamins, minerals, enzymes, trace elements, etc., are necessary to destroy free-radicals. Supplementation of isolated parts has minimal benefit. This points out why nutrition must be correct, and why supplementation cannot work by itself.

The only substance for neutralizing oxygen free-radicals (pollution, tobacco smoke, etc.), however, seems to be beta carotene. This explains why it is associated with reducing risk of cancer. Vitamin E's only function may be to intercept free-radicals and reduce them to a non-toxic form. This may explain the benefits of taking vitamin E supplements. Cholesterol also is a potent anti-oxidant.

* * * * *

Coso healing clay, which is Montmorillonite green type clay, can be very beneficial for many problems. It has formed over millions of years and has been hydrothermally altered by the hot water of volcanic activity, which gives it a negative electrical charge that increases its drawing effect and healing ability.

We are exposed to over 70,000 known and untested chemicals. Toxins accumulate in the colon and the tissues. Coso clay pulls out debris, parasites, and accumulated toxins from the colon. Clay has been used for centuries for ulcers and diarrhea. Combined with psyllium seed it will cause an intestinal cleansing when taken for three to thirty days.

Cats with leukemia are definitely helped with daily doses of clay mixed in water. Maybe people with leukemia would be too.

106

When clay is taken orally its intense activity eliminates and destroys unhealthy cells, and activates rebuilding (colloidal). It is cleansing, it purifies and enriches the blood, and acts as a catalyst by rebuilding tissue and cells. Clay absorbs radioactivity, and awakens energy resources which normally remain dormant. It has organo-therapeutic value, and is rich in enzymes. Its effect can be truly remarkable! Although somewhat difficult to find, perhaps your local health food store will order it for you. Highly recommended for digestive problems, ulcers, liver problems, gallbladder problems, and general improvement of health because of detoxification and enzymes.

Pascalite, one of the best healing clays, mined in the Big Horn mountains of Wyoming, can be ordered from the Pendergraft's at Box 104, 1220 Pulliam Ave., Worland, Wyoming 82401, or call (307) 347-3872.

* * * * *

Animals can be helped, sometimes immensely, with the following natural approaches. From experience I know that veterinarians are usually against this, and in some cases will, instead, let them die or prescribe expensive, worthless treatments.

If your dog or cat has seizures give them calcium-magnesium-zinc and/or pau d'arco. If they have tumors pau d'arco will cause them to disappear -- dissolve or breakup, or disrupt through the skin. Fasting two days may cause tumors to disappear, also. Enzymes may help many sicknesses, as will fasting and vitamins.

If your cat has leukemia give them high potency vitamin C, multiple vitamins with minerals, and pau d'arco. Try germanium. Your cat will live much longer and more comfortably than with veterinarian/chemical-drug treatment. I've tried both ways, unfortunately for little Sabrina and fortunately for Louie. And last, but not least, use Montmorillonite clay. Either put the clay/water mixture on them to lick off, or put it in their mouth. The germanium or clay approaches may have astounding results after a week or two. Also, Co-enzyme Q10 has been proven to help animals with tumors and leukemia.

If your cat has feline infectious peritonitis give high potency vitamin C, multiple vitamins with minerals, and high potency garlic to lessen the water retention in the stomach, or chest. It may be the germanium in the garlic which relieves fluid retention. Therefore, germanium tablets may be helpful.

If animals have heart problems give them high potency vitamin E once a week, and garlic daily to lower blood pressure.

If they're constipated, give at least a tablespoon of psyllium powder daily. Remember, a cat's metabolism is about seven times faster than a human's. So is a dog's. So they need about the amount an adult human would need.

Skin problems and ear problems are helped with vitamin E, or garlic, applied topically. Old age problems are countered with calcium-magnesium-zinc, high potency vitamin C, alfalfa, enzymes, and salmon oil.

Look at the ingredients in the processed food for your animals. Some of them are beyond bad. Replace their old diet with at least some natural diet. Read *The New Natural Cat* by Anitra Frazier. This is a very comprehensive medical book for natural approaches to health for your cat, and has many dietary suggestions.

A wonderfully effective broth for many health problems is cabbage, potatoes, garlic (a lot), parsley (a lot), onion, celery and its leaves (a lot), carrots, and broccoli. Cover with water, and simmer one half hour. Give broth for 1 to 2 days, possibly alternating with other food. Healthy cats will like the vegetables, so don't throw them away if you have other cats! They need green vegetables at least once a week.

Like people, cats need natural nutrients and sometimes supplementary vitamins and minerals. "Pet Tinic" -- an iron, B-vitamin, copper supplement is highly recommended.

Sick animals need extra vitamin and mineral supplementation, with potassium. The broth above provides all of these, especially potassium, in a natural form. A good mixture that can also be given to cats needing to be fed by syringe is raw egg, clay, Willard Water (mixed with water), psyllium powder, dissolved high potency vitamins and minerals, and that same vegetable broth. Willard Water (mixed with water) should be used 1 teaspoon to a gallon (not the human dose), and be given daily for possibly wonderful results! Note: Use three quarters of a teaspoon to a gallon if on medicine, because it enhances the action of medication.

DMSO, a mineral product in powder form, is available from feed stores. It is very safe and effective for animals. (Follow directions.)

Essiac, from Wow-Bow distributors, may be the best of all. It eliminated tumors from one of my young cats, and restored my chronically ill 12 year old cat to greatly improved health and energy.

A famous veterinarian who uses a holistic approach is Dr. Pitcairn, author of a book called *Dr. Pitcairn's*

Complete Guide to Natural Health for Dogs and Cats.
It is highly recommended.

The Natural Pet Care Products Catalog, from Washington, is free at 1-800-962-8266. Wow-Bow Healthy Alternatives Catalog for Pets is free at 1-800-326-0230.

* * * * *

In one of the most comprehensive drinking water studies the Natural Resources Defense Council analyzed EPA records and found that in 1991 and 1992 43% of all water supplies in the United States violated Federal health standards. There were 250,000 violations affecting more than 120 million people. State and Federal regulators, however, acted on just 3,900 of the 250,000 violations. Non community water systems (hospitals, hotels, and schools) had an added 10,000 violations affecting 1.4 million people.

Bacteria, viruses, and cysts like cryptosporidium sicken about a million people a year, and kill about 1000 a year (NRDC). A survey by the Center for Disease Control showed that in 1989 and 1990 4288 people in 16 states got sick from these pathogens, and four died.

About 10,000 new bladder and rectal cancer cases per year are caused by trihalomethanes, which are by-products of chloride (NRDC) (chlorination).

Excess lead in drinking water causes high blood pressure, behavior problems, hypertension, and nerve damage. Exposure to lead levels, in general, are *3000--6000%* higher now than those of pre-industrial humans, according to the U.S. Department of Health.

110

The Environmental Protection Agency chief Carol Browner said, "The way we guarantee safe drinking water is broken and needs to be fixed." Over 2,100 chemicals in U.S. water supplies need to be removed and/or regulated. Less than 2% of violations are acted upon by regulators.

Consumer Reports revealed one of the best systems for removal of lead and chemicals was developed by a company called Multi-Pure that uses a solid carbon block. This is the most advanced and effective technology in instant water filtration, reducing chlorine, asbestos, cysts, lead, pesticides, turbidity, and 20 volatile organic chemicals. It doesn't remove minerals, like distilled water does. It also reduces or eliminates trihalomethanes, lindane, and 2.4-D. To get information about Multi-Pure call 1-800-656-9399.

Joseph Price, M.D., in his book *Coronaries, Cholesterol, and Chlorine* offers proof that chlorine is a major cause of coronaries and strokes, not cholesterol. He lists non-toxic alternatives to chlorine, which he proves is not necessary to purify drinking water.

Effects of water fluoridation are completely researched in *Fluoride: The Aging Factor* by John Yiamouyiannis, Ph.D. He reports damage to bones and teeth, premature aging, arthritis, cancer, and death caused by fluoride in toothpaste, dental treatments, and in water.

Clean, high quality water is essential to better health and a better life.

* * * * *

Catalyst Altered Willard Water has some very unusual properties. Benefits include reduction of stress, reduction of swelling, greatly increased absorption of nutrients, more efficient elimination of wastes and toxins, and it works as an anti-oxidant and scavenger of free-radicals. It was patented about 15 years ago. It helps the body heal itself. Results can be amazing.

By using the Catalyst Altered Water the valuable and needed nutrients that have been locked up in lignite for millions of years are now made available to man. Dr. Willard experimented for over twenty years before being able to successfully extract nutrients, trace minerals, humic acids, and amino acids from lignite, found in coal deposits. Lignite is the fossil remains of plants that grew during and before the Age of Dinosaurs.

Carbon can be changed into a diamond or a pencil simply by rearranging its molecular structure. It is much the same with Willard Water because the catalyst micelle is added to regular water and alters the molecular structure of the water. Changing a substance's structure changes its properties. So diamonds are extremely hard, but graphite (pencil lead) is extremely soft.

Beware of substitutes and imitations. They don't work. A legitimate source is: Dakota Providers at P.O. Box 8023, Fargo, North Dakota 58109-8023. Or, call them at 1-800-447-4793.

* * * * *

Natural sea salt can rejuvenate the body's bio-system. It is a remedy for many health problems. No pill supplement equals the minerals that natural sea salt supplies. It has reversed chronic illness. Because of its complex beneficial minerals and bio-electronic power it offers many health benefits, such as restoring acid/alkaline levels, good digestion, allergy relief, and elimination of skin diseases. Also, increased energy, resistance to infections and bacterial diseases.

If a natural and better diet is started in order to heal, it should include natural, unrefined Celtic salt. The absence of salt in the daily diet greatly hampers absorption of nutrients contained in grains and vegetables, making them unable to function as natural healing agents.

An acidic body condition is at the root of many sicknesses. Since Celtic seasalt alkalinizes, it is a remedy. The body requires extra potassium when there is hemorrhaging, severe burns, physical trauma, acute infection, emotional turmoil, or shock from illness or surgery. This is best done with salt in water. (Sodium transmutes to potassium.) Celtic seasalt is the best salt to maintain optimum health.

Our bodies contain three internal fluids that require frequent mineral replenishment of many trace elements, best accomplished by taking minute amounts of salt in our food. These fluids are blood plasma, lymphatic circulatory system fluids, and extracellular fluid. These body fluids influence one another. This explains why a variation of the external environment -- heat, humidity, electromagnetic forces -- and internal environment variations -- diet, acidity, etc., -- has such a definite bearing on the body's whole internal self.

Seasalts possess therapeutic qualities capable of restoring balance, even in long-standing chronic problems. Trace elements work together to maintain proper functioning of body systems.

All medical and scientific studies condemning salt examined refined white salt -- a biologically damaging, completely unnatural, and chemicalized substance. In the industrialized refining process 82 trace minerals and nutrients are removed, leaving a single compound of sodium and chlorine. Magnesium, bromine, sulfur, etc. are then a great source of profit for the multi-national big ocean chemical business.

Most diets, especially vegetarian and grain diets, require slightly more salt to prevent an excess of sodium over potassium. If this happens the body's enzyme pathway cannot produce hydrochloric acid, an absolutely essential digestive secretion.

A natural food company called Gold Mine has Celtic sea salt, and many other organic products. Call 1-800-475-3663 for a free catalog.

*****

The Peruvian rainforest has herbs that have been used by indigenous cultures for hundreds, even thousands, of years. Countries throughout the world have validated the benefits of many herbs from the rainforest. Jesus told the Essenes: "Purify your blood with herbs, and all things will fall away."

Uncaria tomentosa, or una de gato, is probably one of the best and most useful herbs. It helps cancer, arthritis, painful joints, bursitis, rheumatism, the side effects of chemotherapy, genital herpes, stress, sleep problems, depression, allergies, ulcers, candidiasis, PMS, cycle

114

irregularities, toxin poisoning, AIDS, HIV, bowel and stomach and intestinal disorders, and tumors and growths.

It has a remarkable ability to cleanse the entire intestinal tract. It helps Crohn's disease, diverticulitis, leaky bowel syndrome, hypoglycemia, colitis, hemorrhoids, fistulas, gastritis, parasites, and restores intestinal flora imbalance. It appears to surpass all other herbs and shark cartilage in its ability to heal and build the immune system. It greatly enhances emotional stability.

A Peruvian doctor successfully treated 700 cancer patients, having 14 types of cancer, with una de gato.

It has the potential to stop and reverse deep-seated pathology. It is anti-viral, anti-tumor, anti-inflammatory, anti-free-radical, and anti-oxidant. Truly a wonderful herb!

Illumination is a combination of 33 Amazon rainforest herbs, including una de gato. People have reported wonderful improvements in health after taking it.

Una de gato activates T-lymphocytes and macrophages, which are the body's defense mechanisms. It regulates blood sugar levels very effectively.

Both can be ordered from Rainforest Bio-Energetics in Florida. Call 1-800-835-0850 for more information.

* * * * *

Chronic inflammation results from an excess production of substances produced because of injuries. Tissue damage is the long-term result. Circuma longa, also known as turmeric (seasoning spice), controls these excess substances. It lessens stiffness, swelling, and pain.

115

Imbalances anywhere in the body are normalized by a tonic formerly called Essiac tea, now called Flor•essence. In 1920, a Canadian nurse was given this tonic by a woman whose breast cancer had been healed forty years earlier by an Ojibway medicine man with this remedy. Naturally, the medical establishment has not acknowledged it because it's a natural remedy, etc. It is therefore trademarked as a "food," despite its history of saving lives when nothing else could be done.

Chamomile tea stops insomnia and stress. Bananas and yogurt contain tryptophan, a natural relaxant. Bananas are also natural antacids.

Comfrey tea stimulates tissue regeneration. It is known as "knit-bone." Healing of bone, fractures, muscles, tendon and ligament injuries is a benefit of drinking this tea.

Echinacea greatly helps the immune system. It may eliminate sore throats, flu, infections, allergies, tumors, and it purifies the bloodstream. It grows in the United States and is used extensively in Europe.

Valerian relieves stress, insomnia, and migraine headaches.

Kelp helps combat radiation effects that result in leukemia, bone cancer, anemia, and Hodgkin's disease. It also stabilizes the thyroid.

St. John's wort is good for wounds and to regenerate damaged nerve tissue.

Willard Water heals external wounds and infections very well. Apply in diluted form. (1 ounce added to 1 gallon of water.)

Cranberry juice maintains the health of, and eliminates problems of, the urinary tract, bladder, and kidneys.

One tablespoon of flaxseed oil a day may prevent asthma attacks. Use 1500 mg. of pantothenic acid (B5) for asthma, also.

Natural fat burners are CoQ10 and chromium picolinate.

Maitake mushrooms inhibit tumor growth and help high blood pressure, diabetes, obesity, cancer, HIV, AIDS, and lower cholesterol levels. They have been used for thousands of years.

Hyperbaric Oxygen Treatment provides oxygen to injured cells and decreases swelling of brain tissue. Stroke patients experience up to 100% recovery from paralysis, mental impairment, and other effects of stroke.

*****

Lemon is the best fruit. It is a blood purifier, it tones the heart, cleanses the liver, lessens high blood pressure, helps badly circulating blood, relieves congestion, aids digestion because of the biliary reaction it stimulates, eliminates toxins in the bladder and kidneys (including those that have crystallized), and may help arthritis and rheumatism. Gandhi always drank lemon juice when he was fasting. Lemon dissolves and eliminates. When you're sick, drink a mixture of hot lemon juice, honey, and water.

Cinnamon can cause a 400% improvement in blood sugar regulation in human tissue, thereby influencing diabetes and hypoglycemia.

Brewer's yeast is rich in nucleic acid, a basic element in cell development believed to retard aging. It is the best source of chromium (glucose tolerance factor), which is essential for the production of functionally effective insulin, without which the body cannot properly handle glucose, its major fuel. Brewer's yeast is also rich in selenium, potassium, vitamins, and lecithin. It is the best source for B-complex vitamins, and all the essential amino acids (proteins). It gives energy, and a sense of well-being, helping many health problems. It also helps prevent hair loss.

Ginkgo biloba is used for asthma, edema, and Alzheimer's.

Ginseng and valerian help heart disease. The average heart beats 100,000 times a day, and pumps about 2,000 gallons of blood daily. Decongestants can cause rapid heartbeat. Risk of heart attack increases three times after a hysterectomy.

Allantoin is a natural and ancient healer found in sugar beets. Burns of any severity are helped, sometimes immensely, by allantoin applications. As a matter of fact, applying sugar itself over a burn causes healing to accelerate, apparently because of its inhibition of harmful bacterial multiplication. Also, egg whites and yogurt help heal and stop pain.

Psoriasis is a chronic skin condition of unknown origin marked by red lesions of the skin -- often treated by ultraviolet light. To keep it under control, or eliminate its appearance, take a minimum of 500 mg. vitamin C daily. Also, flaxseed oil (1000 mg.) and ginseng help. Camphor, salicylic acid or willow bark, applied topically, will also help.

Cholesterol is manufactured by every cell in the body. You cannot *live* without it. If you eat more than needed you will synthesize less. If you eat less than you need your body will synthesize more. The body overproduces cholesterol for protection from pollution, poor diet and lack of exercise. It is a potent antioxidant, therefore necessary. To insure proper levels the cause of the problem of excess cholesterol needs to be eliminated. As an example, whole egg yolks are a source of good and beneficial cholesterol. But egg yolks that are broken/scrambled are sources of oxidized cholesterol, which is harmful.

Dr. Julian Whitaker estimated that over 56 million people suffer from cholesterol blockage in legs and heart arteries. Choline dissolves cholesterol deposits in arteries and blood vessels. A good source of choline is lecithin. Vitamin C and choline make cholesterol more soluble so that gallstones are less likely to be formed. Or, they can dissolve existing gallstones. Fiber traps cholesterol and eliminates it from the body. EFA's normalize and balance cholesterol levels. Cholesterol lowering drugs cause a 20% increase in mortality. The nutritional approach is safer and better.

*****

Back surgery is appropriate for less than 10% of chronic back pain patients. Exercise strengthens injured bones and muscles. Take calcium-magnesium-zinc daily to alleviate pain and speed repair. The most effective remedy is daily simple exercise and avoidance of any activity that causes pain. Lower back pain can indicate a need for manganese.

Did you know that the mercury in dental amalgam (fillings) causes illness, kidney problems, cancer, and Alzheimer's? Many studies have proven this to be true. The EPA says mercury is a deadly, toxic substance, so why do dentists put it in our mouths? *Beating Alzheimer's*, by Tom Warren, is enlightening.

Yogurt will stop diarrhea if eaten exclusively for 24 hours.

Altoids are strong peppermints from England, found in grocery stores and drug stores, packaged in small tin containers. They are remarkably effective for ulcer discomfort, esophageal spasms, irritable bowel, and indigestion.

Peppermint concentrate (oil or powder) can have a dramatic effect on health problems. Like all other natural forms of healing the process may take up to six months. It dissolves blood clots, improves circulation and varicose veins. It can gradually restore eyesight. Peppermint helps irregular or painful menstruation and stomach and intestinal ailments; strengthens the heart muscle and nerves; dissolves kidney stones; corrects edema and respiratory tract problems (asthma, colds, flu, infections, etc.); helps liver and gallbladder problems; stops insomnia and ulcers, and cures many other ills. It improves digestion because it reduces stomach acidity and stimulates secretion of bile ten times.

Orthodox doctors do not treat through diet or strengthening the immune system, so the underlying disease remains dormant. It may erupt and spread throughout the body again. As an example, acne can be caused by excess toxic materials overloading the kidneys, liver, bowel and lungs, and is forced to exit through skin as bacteria. This blocks the sebaceous glands and bacteria builds on the skin. Acne medication can cause imbalances of insulin, hormones, or blood pressure. All antibiotics destroy both good and bad bacteria, which can lead to candidas albicans or fungus infection. Therefore, fasting and the Best Diet is a simple, yet often more effective and safe, remedy for acne. Once acne medication is stopped the acne often reoccurs, sometimes worse than before. It is important for the immune system that regular detoxification take place. A juice fast is effective. The body literally burns up only substances that are not needed, that are diseased, or damaged. As these wastes are expelled dramatic changes can occur.

* * * * *

In March of 1993 I experienced my first ordeal with a gallbladder attack. The stone moving through the bile duct causes extreme pain that usually starts between two and four in the morning, and lasts for about two hours. Time for a gallbladder operation, right? Not necessarily. A huge scar, a lot of pain during recuperation, and only about a 75% chance of eliminating the problem were not good alternatives, in my estimation. But the attacks are probably more painful than the surgery and recuperation. Through trial and error and lots of research, which eventually resulted in a chapter about natural solutions to health problems, I found effective ways to avoid this happening again. However, I did have three more gallstone attacks during my time of experimentation. A sonogram revealed they had been passed after the last of these excruciating episodes in March of 1994.

Major indigestion accompanies a gallbladder problem. Gallbladder attacks, and biliary colic, often happen after a heavy meal, or a rich assortment of food. Eating only fruit, vegetables, or juice, that are fresh and raw so you get the enzymes for digestion, works wonders. Also whole grain bread and cereal with no preservatives. And brown rice.

To eat no meat and no food with anything artificial in it means most food in the grocery store can't be tolerated. Accepting a change in eating can be a problem for most people. But understand that this change is necessary to *avoid* many health problems slowly developing in each one of us. The food in any grocery store is what causes a lot of health problems, now or later. So where does one go to find organic food, produced on soil that is rich with natural nutrients, instead of depleted?

Inadequate enzymes in your system are a cause for indigestion. Cooking above 118° F kills enzymes that occur naturally. Avoid indigestion and you'll probably avoid a gallbladder attack. To do this eliminate processed, cooked, and artificial food. No additives, no preservatives, etc. Also, don't eat after about 6:00 at night so there's no undigested food in your system when you go to bed.

Try a juice fast for three days. Fresh juice made with fresh fruit is best. Otherwise try to find unheated, nothing added, juice. Drink as much as you want. Or, try a three to five day grapefruit fast.

Bromelain (enzymes) tablets are a wonderful solution to indigestion. They also help your heart by decreasing chances of blood clots in your arteries, like aspirin is supposed to do. Bromelain is the natural vs. the artificial approach. Take a 100 mg. tablet before each meal.

Papaya enzyme tablets, or Wobenzymes from Germany, may work even better. Experiment. Either one takes about half an hour to be effective. Lactobacillus acidophilus taken before meals is very beneficial, too. Hydrochloric acid is absolutely necessary for digestion-- supplements may be necessary, especially if you're over 35. Niacin and Celtic sea salt help produce HCL.

If you feel a problem coming on take a brisk walk for 20 to 30 minutes. Or, take strong Altoids mints from England to counteract indigestion. As many as 5 to 10 may be necessary.

Taking at least 2400 grams of lecithin, capsules or liquid, daily is supposed to dissolve the stones. Cholesterol gallstones are dissolved by vitamin C and choline (in lecithin). Pure lemon juice is also supposed to dissolve them, and drinking it helps anyone feel better. Both approaches seemed to work for me. Also, dandelion stems dissolve gallstones.

These have been my most successful solutions to avoid recurrences of gallbladder problems. Having your gallbladder removed does not eliminate the reasons the stones developed in the first place. Lack of free-flowing bile can be remedied by not eating food that bothers you (an allergic reaction), by drinking 6 to 8 glasses of pure water daily, by taking lipotromic formulas which include betaine hydrochloride (HCL), avoiding fat, taking milk thistle (silymarin) capsules, and drinking nettle tea.

There is a purpose for every part of the human body. To remove them may upset some balance that can't be regained. Doctors say there is no need for the uterus after child bearing years so take it out. This cavalier attitude has influenced doctors to remove millions of women's uteruses. The side effects are increase of heart attacks, increase of cholesterol, an increased need for fiber in the diet, and a need to replace hormones indefinitely. And an increase in breast cancer. Natural menopause shuts down the ovaries, reducing estrogen, progesterone, and androgen production by about 50%. Total hysterectomies reduce hormone output 100% because they remove the ovaries with the uterus -- a radical and traumatic physical, emotional, spiritual change for

123

women.   A struggle to restore homeostasis, balance, results. What balance is upset permanently by removal of the gallbladder?

* * * * *

My daughter had a big problem for years with allergies of unknown origins.   After several three day (sometimes longer) modified fasting sessions (juice, etc.) over a period of about five months, the very aggravating symptoms vastly improved.   Actually, they improved greatly after the first modified juice fast, but came back with a vengeance after resuming usual eating habits. So, modified fasts are helpful for her every month or two. They probably would be helpful, too, for the millions of other people who also suffer from allergies. Try it, you'll like the results.

My neighbor burned her finger very badly on microwaved pizza cheese.   After she returned from her doctor I told her to take 1000 to 1500 milligrams (mg.) of vitamin C every day, 500 mg. each time, 2 to 3 times daily. She did, and her doctor remarked later that her finger had healed amazingly well and fast. It certainly had!

* * * * *

Vitamins and minerals are essential to health. Some health problems can be helped, or alleviated, with extra amounts of appropriate minerals and vitamins. Some health problems can be prevented.

124

Minerals help create cell energy. To maintain or regain health a correction of mineral deficiencies, or improper assimilation, is necessary to produce a saliva or urine Ph ("potential hydrogen") level of 6.4. It doesn't matter what the illness is, what the name of it is. We just need to correct the imbalance. Balanced body chemistry enables the body to heal itself.

Vitamin C promotes feeling better, increases energy, heals and stops psoriasis, helps urinary tract, kidney, and bladder problems. It is water soluble so regular replacement is essential. It maintains collagen and heals wounds, burns, and surgical cuts, because it facilitates formation of connective tissue. It fights infection and reduces the effects of some allergies. I know from personal experience that vitamin C does, indeed, do all these things by taking at least two 500 mg. tablets once or twice a day. Vitamin C also destroys nitrates, a cancer-causing agent in food. For cancer take four or five grams daily (1000 mg. = 1 gram). Absorption of vitamin C is improved by several smaller dosages daily, instead of one large dose, because it stays in your system for only about 12 hours. Also, vitamin C helps avoid and alleviate anemia and Alzheimer's disease, and stops or slows the progression of the HIV virus.

Nobel Peace Prize winner Linus Pauling wrote a book about cancer and using vitamin C in its treatment. Cancer is caused by agents or conditions which change the genetic material of the cells. Vitamin C seems to protect the cells. He determined that, in fact, vitamin C is one of the most important vitamins in the prevention and treatment of cancer. Also, it protects the heart, increases resistance to infections, protects eyes, teeth, gums, cells, and blood vessels.

Vitamin A reduces susceptibility to infections, helps maintain a smooth, soft skin, and helps growth and repair of tissues. Beta carotene is a precursor of vitamin A found naturally in yellow, orange, and dark green fruit and vegetables. Doctor's studies involving thousands of people have revealed that 50 mg. of beta carotene daily reduces heart attacks, strokes, and deaths related to heart disease, by about one-half. It is essential for health of bones, skin, hair, teeth, and gums.

Vitamin E slows or reverses fatty build-up on arterial walls, contributing thereby to a healthy heart. It may protect against cancer and heart disease. It enhances immunity, retards formation of cataracts, promotes good circulation, protects red blood cells, and is essential to the health of skin, reproductive organs, and muscles. It can have a dramatic effect on the reproductive organs, and prevents miscarriages. It is an anti-oxidant that prevents accumulation of free-radicals. It increases endurance and prevents aging, scar formation, and damage from pollution. It helps complexion problems, high blood pressure, and heart problems. Also, skin cancer, tumors, and breast cancer. Use 400 mg., never more than 800 mg., because it accumulates in the body.

All B vitamins are water soluble. An excess is therefore impossible -- it would be discharged. They are very important for health of nerves, and metabolism and energy. High potencies greatly help nervous, tense people, and also cancer patients in chemotherapy. The best source of all B and high potency B vitamins is in brewer's yeast. Within a week of taking it you should feel better, look better, have an improved complexion, and increased energy. It doesn't taste too good, but it's worth it!

Vitamins are constituents of enzymes. Enzymes function as catalysts in metabolic reactions. So vitamins help regulate metabolism. They also convert fat and carbohydrates into energy, and assist in bone and tissue formation. Vitamins are incapable of working without minerals. They work synergistically with each other.

An organ with a low blood supply recovers slowly. An organ with a high blood supply recovers more quickly because more enzymes are available to digest the disease, illness, cancer, or tumor. For this purpose vitamins are important because they are co-enzymes. Enzymes need co-enzymes. And minerals activate the enzyme/co-enzyme reactions. They all need each other.

A U. S. D. A. study determined 90% of Americans have a chromium deficiency because of processed foods, refined sugar, soda pop, and deficiency in the soils. Chromium is a co-factor of insulin. It helps convert sugar into energy. A deficiency means the body cannot convert sugar into energy so it stores the excess as fat. It aids in controlling sugar levels, and the production of insulin used in the breakdown of sugar in the body, and hormone balance. It also lowers cholesterol.

Chromium picolinate is a very bioactive source of this essential mineral. It helps to control appetite and sugar cravings, and helps prevent loss of muscle and organ tissue that results from low calorie diets.

According to a U.S. Senate study (Document #264), 99% of Americans are deficient in all minerals and trace elements. Why? Because of over-processed foods and depleted soil, over-planted and saturated with synthetic fertilizers and pesticides. Supplementation is therefore necessary to prevent premature aging, to stay healthy, to ward off cancer and heart disease.

All bodily processes depend on the action and presence of minerals. Vitamins cannot function without minerals. Minerals are needed for healing and tissue rebuilding. This explains why soaking in water heals wounds. Minerals are difficult to absorb. As an example, both calcium and iron are better absorbed with vitamin C. Mineral supplements need to be water soluble, and taken with vitamins, in order to provide maximum benefit.

Our cells contain more potassium than any other mineral. Potassium influences nerve transmission, muscle contraction, and hormone secretion.

Calcium with magnesium and zinc helps avoid age related bone loss, reduces hip fractures and non vertebral fractures, and lowers blood pressure. It helps eliminate bone and muscle pain, arthritis discomfort, bone spurs, and sometimes seizures. Zinc helps acne and other skin problems, encourages healthy hair growth, and prevents hair loss and wrinkles. Calcium must have magnesium and vitamin D to be assimilated.

Fifteen minutes of daily exposure to the sun will give anyone enough vitamin D for that day.

Selenium may protect against cancer, enhances the effectiveness of vitamin E, and preserves tissue elasticity.

Beta carotene (or vitamin A), vitamin C, vitamin E, and selenium are the anti-oxidant vitamins. They control and minimize free-radical reactions within the cell. They inactivate dangerous free-radical reactions which contribute to aging and ill-health. Free-radicals are highly reactive, unstable compounds that are formed each day through normal body processes. Free-radical precursors are formed by radiation, pollution, cigarette smoke, and herbicides. Free-radicals can cause severe damage to cell structures resulting in premature internal aging, so these vitamins prolong youth and health.

However, it is not enough to use food supplements. The organism must be brought to a condition where it can extract what it needs from food in its natural form. The liver must be in good working order. When food is natural, and the liver is accomplishing its normal work, deficiencies are taken care of without any intervention. A diet reinforced with many vitamin supplements may only aggravate the situation by making the liver overactive. Absorption and retention of vitamins and minerals in supplements can be a problem because they are highly refined, and/or chemically produced. This is especially true if the liver is dysfunctional. Plant substances and herbs, however, are easily assimilated. It is preferable, therefore, to use natural vitamins instead of synthetic.

*****

A larger percentage of our nation's population is over 65 years of age than ever before. Along with aging comes health problems. Many of these common problems can be helped or alleviated with natural solutions.

The environmental movement now understands that preservation of entire ecosystems is preferable to the preservation of individual species. This more intelligent approach to wildlife correlates with the preservation of human health. The entire body or system's health needs to be preserved and supported, instead of just attending to separate illnesses/problems.

Joint trouble is one of the major causes of suffering because of aging. Millions of people have constant pain and stiffness. Anti-inflammatory medication may actually speed the degenerative process of joints, but glucosamine sulfate relieves the pain and restores healthy joint tissue. This natural compound stimulates production of joint-rebuilding mucopolysaccharides, restores normal cartilage, and reverses the process of degeneration. Relief of discomfort and increased mobility are possible naturally, reversing the underlying cause.

CoQ10 is found naturally in the body, but tissue levels diminish as we grow older. The result is less energy, more health problems, less vitality. CoQ10 keeps tissues and organs functioning at maximum efficiency, and helps detoxify the body. Also, at least 300 mg. daily have eliminated tumors.

Most men over the age of 60 experience prostate problems. Saw palmetto and zinc can protect against this, or help alleviate it once it has begun.

Many of the well-known signs of aging can be counteracted with ginkgo biloba. It naturally improves blood flow to the brain and extremities by dilating blood vessels. The result is more energy, better memory, better mood, and mental clarity.

Vitamin C (1000 mg.) and a multiple vitamin-mineral supplement are other insurances against aging too fast. Ginseng, una de gato, aloe, and Willard Water all have the desired ability to *balance* an imbalanced body/system. Therefore, all of these supplements may counteract and slow the process of aging. Unlike pharmaceuticals, all of these supplements, as described, have no side effects and are completely safe for senior citizens.

* * * * *

Causes of mental problems can be toxicity, allergies, nutritional imbalances and deficiencies. Mental stress often results in physical problems. Emotional health and physical health are closely related. The Chinese believe that if you heal your mind the body will follow.

There are ways to combat stress and depression naturally. Light activity (gardening, shopping, etc.) makes a person happier. (Each hour of activity may add one and a half hours to your life.) Set goals and reach them. Make friends and socialize. Daylight, sunlight, is essential to the physical and mental health of everyone. To avoid depression make time to be outdoors. Also, use ginkgo biloba, high potency B-complex vitamins, ginseng, or una de gato to eliminate depression and stress.

* * * * *

We are all the same physiologically, but we are all different physiologically. Unique, but not unique. That's why treatments for health problems often need to be individualized, tailored to the individual. That's why prevention programs work for some people and not for others.

Use nutritional therapy for physiological imbalances. Also, for many psychological problems that instead may be nutritional imbalances.

A list of natural, alternative solutions to common health problems follows. A natural diet and inner cleansing (detoxification) is the first step for each problem. Exercise, vitamin-mineral-enzyme supplementation, no meat or sugar or coffee/caffeine, no chemicals, no additives, pertain to all.

Digestion problems --   Enzymes (at least 400 mg. daily)
                         Garlic
                         Niacin
                         Algae (has 300% more oxygen
                             than alfalfa)
                         Additional fiber
                         Lactobacillus acidophilus
                         Herbal combinations for
                             candida albicans
                         Altoids peppermints
                         Hydrochloric acid (HCL)
                         Celtic sea salt
                         Lemon juice
                         Una de gato

Candida Albicans --   Astralagus
                         Garlic
                         Pau d'arco
                         Una de gato
                         Herbal combinations for yeast
                             infections

Chronic Fatigue --   Pau d'arco
                         Una de gato
                         Brewer's yeast
                         Enzymes
                         Vitamin C
                         Herbs for candida albicans
                         Betaine HCL
                         Lecithin
                         Essiac tea
                         Ginseng

Multiple Sclerosis & Parkinson's disease --	Yarrow tea Sage tea Essiac tea Grape seed extract Swedish bitters
Weight Loss --	Chromium Bromelain Co Q10 EFA's Brewer's yeast Evening primrose oil
Gallstones & Gallbladder problems --	Lecithin Swedish bitters Lemon juice Dandelion tea and stems Enzymes Minerals Avoid rich food Avoid dairy products Drink more water Betaine HCL Milk thistle (silymarin) Nettle tea
Asthma --	Flax oil (1 tablespoon) daily Eliminate chemicals A juice fast Ginseng Herbs for candida albicans Ginkgo biloba Pantothenic acid (B5) 1500 mg.

Insomnia or PMS -- Candida herb combinations
Una de gato
Essential Fatty Acids
Pau d'arco
Valerian
Chamomile tea
Rosemary tea

Hormone imbalances -- Ginseng
Yucca
Fennel
Black cohosh herbs
Mexican yams
Vitamin E (400 IU)
Candida herb combinations
Una de gato
Pyridoxine (vitamin B6).
Milk thistle
Sarsaparilla

Pain -- Feverfew
Swedish bitters

Prostate Problems -- Saw palmetto
Vitamin D
Zinc
Flaxseed oil (1000 mg.)

Depression or
Stress -- SEE ALZHEIMER'S
SEE ALZHEIMER'S

High Cholesterol or High Blood Pressure --	Garlic Calcium-magnesium-zinc Co Q10 Una de gato Ginseng Yucca Dandelion Vitamin C (1000 mg.) Black cohosh herbs Gum guggulow herbs Lemon juice
Hypoglycemia --	Manganese Vitamin C Siberian ginseng Chromium picolinate Brewer's yeast
Alzheimer's --	Magnesium/calcium Kelp Chamomile Ginkgo biloba Co Q10 Ginseng Algae Alfalfa Superoxide dismatuse (SoD) EFA's Una de gato Candida combinations (herbs) Eliminate mercury (amalgam fillings) EDTA (amino acid)

Joint problems --	Co Q10
	Anti-oxidants like SoD
	Niacin (100 mg.)
	Glucosamine sulfate
	Minerals
	Nettle tea
	Swedish bitters
Behavior problems and Hyperactivity --	A juice fast
	Vitamin/mineral supplements
	No chemicals
	Exercise
	No meat
	Valerian
	Grapeseed extract
A Depressed/Debilitated Immune System --	Oatmeal
	Bran
	Apples
	No meat (to clear fat and cholesterol from the blood and blood vessels)
	Co Q10
	SEE ALSO " ALLERGIES " LIST
	Echinacea
	Essiac tea (Flor•essence)
	Astralagus
	Una de gato
	Pau d'arco
	Lecithin
	Garlic
	Vitamin C (at least 500 mg.)

Allergies -- Enzymes
Quercetin
Grape seed extract
Organic food
Juice fasts
Bromelain
Una de gato
Ginkgo biloba
Vitamin C (at least 500 mg.)
Pau d'arco
No meat
Celtic sea salt

Psoriasis -- Flaxseed oil
Brewer's yeast
Vitamin C (at least 500 mg.)
Camphor (applied topically)
Willow bark/salicylic acid
(applied topically)

Cancer and
Leukemia -- Co Q10 (large amounts)
Wobenzymes
Flax oil <u>eaten with cottage
cheese or yogurt</u>
Pau d'arco
Una de gato
Algae
EFA's
Alfalfa
Grape seed extract
SoD
Montmorillonite clay
No chemicals

Cancer (continued) --   Vitamin C (at least 4000 mg.)
                        Germanium
                        Shark cartilage or bovine
                          cartilage
                        Haelan 851
                        Essiac tea (Flor•essence)
                        Eliminate mercury (amalgam
                          fillings)
                        No root canals
                        Yarrow tea
                        Calendula tea
                        Nettle tea
                        Calamus tea
                        Bedstraw tea

External cancer --   Castor oil applied topically.

Edema --   Uva ursi (herb)
                        Vitamin B6
                        Ginkgo biloba
                        Milk thistle
                        Willard Water
                        Aloe vera juice

Rheumatism
and/or Arthritis --   Juice fasts
                        Herbal combinations
                        Lemon juice
                        Aloe
                        Co Q10
                        Garlic
                        Yucca tablets
                        Grape seed extract
                        No meat

(continued)-- Calcium-magnesium-zinc
Glucosamine sulfate
Devil's claw
B-complex vitamins -- especially
B6

Heart problems -- Co Q10
Calcium-magnesium-zinc
Vitamin E (400 IU -- 800 IU)
Ginseng
Valerian
Beta carotene (50 mg.)
Vitamin C (1000 mg., or more)
Lecithin
No meat or fat
Garlic
Grape seed extract
EFA's
B-complex vitamins -- especially
B6
Nettle tea
Swedish bitters

It is usually better to work <u>with</u> Nature to improve your health, (the naturopathic and holistic approach), instead of fighting it, (the allopathic approach).

"Natural forces within us are the true
healers of disease."
-- Hippocrates

* * * * *

CHAPTER VIII
HOW TO HAVE NATURAL BEAUTY
AND DELAY AGING

How one looks and presents oneself has a direct effect on career, love life, and self-esteem. It is important to be healthy to fulfill these possibilities. It also helps to use a little assistance that is both cosmetic and naturally derived, instead of chemically derived.

To tighten your complexion and temporarily eliminate wrinkles and sags, put egg white in a little mineral water, mix, and apply. The effect is like expensive creams! For large pores apply a mixture of sesame oil and vitamin C, which is ascorbic acid. To fade scars apply fresh pineapple because bromelain is a natural protein digesting enzyme.

For skin creams mix or use any or all of these: Cod liver oil (has vitamins A and D), allantoin, gelatin (collagen), lanolin oil, olive oil (cold-pressed), aloe, vitamin E, squalene, liposomes, chamomile, peanut oil, hyaluronic acid, beta carotene, royal jelly, and glycerine.

Hyaluronic acid is, perhaps, the most effective humectant. It holds 400 times its weight in water. It's impossible to replace collagen and elastin lost and damaged by free-radicals and ultraviolet rays. But hyaluronic acid creates this effect, increasing firmness and elasticity.

Natural sources of beauty are herbs, vitamins and minerals, and clay -- all applied topically. One of the easiest ways to impart the benefits of minerals onto your skin is with clay. Clays have a high content of minerals. Your skin can readily absorb these minerals during a facial mask treatment. Minerals nourish the skin as they pull impurities from your pores. They regenerate the skin by remineralizing it. Montmorillonite clay from southern France and California contains 50% silica, 12% aluminum oxide, 10% magnesium oxide. Mineral contents vary according to the type of clay. Externally and internally this is the best to use.

These are the best herbal skin beautifiers:

Aloe vera prevents evaporation of moisture, and fights wrinkles and aging skin. It also encourages exfoliation of dead skin and stimulates new cell growth.

Calendula or marigold ward off wrinkles.

Comfrey stimulates new cell growth and strengthens the skin. It contains allantoin and carotene.

Ginseng stimulates, strengthens, rejuvenates, protects, softens, normalizes oily or dry skin, and increases elasticity of the skin.

Rosemary stimulates circulation and acts as a skin rejuvenator that prevents aging.

Chamomile helps acceleration of cell and tissue regeneration.

Jojoba most resembles skin's sebum, so is an excellent moisturizer, and unblocks skin's pores.

Lavender is an excellent skin rejuvenator that balances dry or oily skin. Its calming fragrance eases stress and tension, bringing relaxation.

Glycolic acid, from sugar beets, helps blemishes, clogged pores, wrinkles, scars, and improves skin texture.

Most synthetic ingredients in commercial cosmetics are derived from non-reusable, petro-chemically-derived fossil fuels, creating environmental and personal health problems. Herbal products have been used for thousands of years with no health problems created *anywhere.*

Flax oil is famous for its ability to make skin smooth, velvety soft, and healthy. Ultimate Oil is a combination of flax oil, safflower oil, black currant oil, and vitamin E, to be taken internally for " the glow of youth! " (At least it's a possibility.)

Yucca improves skin problems because of its naturally occurring cortisone. Red clover and colloidal silver help acne.

New You skin rejuvenator uses all natural ingredients to eliminate lines, wrinkles, scars, and brown spots. The result can be truly amazing. For information call 1-800-461-3911.

Dr. Paavo Airola developed "Formula F Plus" many years ago. It is still a great combination. Mix 2 tablespoons sesame oil, 1 tablespoon olive oil, 2 tablespoons avocado oil, 2 tablespoons almond oil, 2000 units vitamin E (mixed tocopherol), 100,000 units vitamin A. This mixture also makes skin velvety smooth and healthy.

Natural humectants like aloe vera or sodium PCA are effective because they pull moisture from the air onto your skin, and keep it there.

Strawberries return your complexion to the proper Ph balance.

Ancient Oriental philosophy believes the aging process shows personal beauty from the inside out. So envy, hate, resentment, and anger will eventually show on anyone's face. I have a very crabby neighbor who is the perfect example of this. The ravages of time, then, become the ravages of the inner self, finally showing itself to the outer world on the face. Hopefully not your face!

Facial massage slows the effects of aging because it uses accupressure and muscle manipulation of involuntary muscles of the face. These muscles get little use, and sag and age sooner. Bringing increased circulation to the mouth and facial muscles will make a woman look younger. Also, complexion improvements and clarity are other benefits.

Apply oils before massaging to reduce stretching and pulling, and improve and maintain elasticity. Cold-pressed olive oil is possibly the best to use for this, and to maintain or create a beautiful complexion.

There are several massage methods to use. One of the best is to tap with the tips of your fingers. Using the fourth finger tap lightly around each eye several times. Using both hands use the tips of four fingers to tap the face. Start at the jawline and tap to the top of your forehead. Do this five to ten times. Then do your neck.

Another method is to use the palms of both hands, working upward only, to lift the muscles. Never pull or tap downward. There's no reason to speed up the aging process!

A company called Tamiko, in Hawaii, sells battery operated face massagers and a massage instruction book, at 1-800-222-4687.

In an article in the Swedish newspaper *Halsoblast* three U.S. movie stars said Vegesil, a silica extract, contributed to their beautiful hair, skin, and nails. The U.S. distributor is Flora, at 1-800-498-3610.

All of these ingredients and methods are safe, natural, and give good -- even great -- results. You'll have to experiment to find your best combinations.

An alternative is to buy environmentally-kind, additive-free, and cruelty-free products from your health food store.

* * * * *

What causes aging? First and foremost, of course, the passage of time. The downward pull of gravity. Chemicals and drugs -- which are poisons. Cigarettes and alcohol -- also poisons. Stress -- which also contributes to various skin disorders, poor health, and diseases. And free-radicals, which are an inevitable fact of life. These highly unstable atoms have unpaired electrons which destroy millions of unhealthy cells. Normally, they are controlled by the immune system, digestion, and metabolism, which rely on free-radicals to initiate chemical reactions. Today's lifestyles generate an excess of free-radicals. Pollution, household chemicals, stress, processed food, saturated fats, pesticides, additives, drugs, cigarette smoke, alcohol, the sun's ultraviolet rays -- all of these generate excessive free-radicals endangering health, and causing premature aging.

Also, oxidation of cell membranes is considered a major factor in aging. Anti-oxidants are found in chamomile, rosemary, ginseng, garlic, ginkgo, and vitamins A, C, E, and selenium. The ginkgo is the only living tree to survive the Ice Age and the atomic blast in Japan. Ginkgo biloba supplements improve blood flow to reduce swelling, stop depression, improve memory and clarity of thinking. Pycnogenol, from the bark of the maritime pine tree, is fifty times stronger than vitamin E, twenty times stronger than vitamin C, as an anti-oxidant. In creams, it returns tissue to a more youthful state. Grapeseed extract is even more effective.

Aging occurs when the hormone system and immune system are functioning inadequately. (Refer to all remedies discussed previously.)

Shortage of oxygen, a primary cause of aging, can be minimized by deep breathing exercises for about fifteen minutes a day. Vitamins A, C, E, and selenium, algae, chlorella, and germanium increase oxygen to the cells, and prevent aging. Wheat germ promotes cell repair and oxygenation.

We each have about one trillion cells. Often, an increased intake of chelated minerals (not organic because they are hard to digest) will prevent cells from premature aging. Mineral imbalance in the tissues is one of the main causes of oxygen shortage, resulting in disease and premature aging. Lack of cellular nourishment causes aging. A solution is fresh, raw organic vegetable or fruit juices, which are rich in minerals.

Vitamin C acts as a support and strengthener of skin. Without this strength and support the skin becomes wrinkled and loose. Besides citrus fruit, cherries are a great source, helping you to have smoother, younger looking skin. Also, vitamin E, 400 to 800 IU's daily, helps a lot.

Fluoride, from any source, causes accelerated aging by breaking down collagen, which makes up about 30% of our body. Weakening of bones, ligaments, muscles, and tendons, and wrinkling of your face are the result.

PABA, in B-complex vitamins (brewer's yeast), returns gray hair to normal, (as does una de gato), makes skin smooth and unwrinkled, and gives energy. Siberian ginseng, chlorella, algae, barley grass, ginkgo biloba, B-complex vitamins, at least 500 mg. vitamin C, una de gato, the Best Diet, detoxification, and exercise are some of the very best ways to delay aging.

* * * * *

145

CHAPTER IX
SOME LEADERS IN ALTERNATIVE HEALTH

Dr. Paavo Airola, a world renowned authority and author of many books, published a book called *How to Get Well* in 1974. This very comprehensive book, covering all aspects of natural healing that are nutritional and drugless, was a bestseller more than twenty years ago.

His basic ideas were that multitudes suffer and die needlessly; that there are simple and effective ways of restoring health (some of them have been used in Europe for many years); that disease is disharmony caused by severe stresses and excesses; and that the primary cause of disease is the weakened organism or lowered resistance, not bacteria. Bacteria is the result of disease, not the cause.

In *How to Get Well* Dr.Airola says:

" The systemic arrangement and biochemical and mctabolic disorder brought about by prolonged physical and mental stresses to which the patient has been subjected -- such as faulty nutritional patterns, constant overeating, overindulgence in proteins and the body's inability to digest them properly, nutritional deficiencies, sluggish metabolism and consequent retention of toxic metabolic wastes, exogenous poisons from polluted food, water, air, and environment, toxic drugs, tobacco and alcohol, lack of sufficient exercise, rest and relaxation, severe emotional and physical stresses, etc. These health destroying environmental factors bring about derangement in all body functions with

146

consequent biochemical imbalance in the
tissues, autotoxemia, chronic undersupply
of oxygen to the cells, poor digestion and
ineffective assimilation of nutrients -- and
gradually lowered resistance to disease. "
(HOW TO GET WELL, Health Plus Publishers, Sherwood, Oregon, 1974.)
This is a perfect description of the problems we all encounter, and of the consequences.

Cure disease and ill health by eliminating the cause. How? Dr. Airola said optimum nutrition, special diets, vitamins and supplements, cleansing (fasting), juices, and herbs. Restore health by removing the causes, by correcting the reason the problem exists, which are health destroying living habits.

You can take charge of your own health and live longer, feel better, and get well. The body can heal itself! Drugs suppress and alleviate symptoms, doing nothing about the cause of the sickness. But nutritional and biological therapies strengthen the body to encourage healing. By strengthening the immune system you strengthen resistance to disease and create the best conditions for the body to heal itself, correcting the underlying cause of disease.

These are naturopathic medical approaches (like an N.D. uses) instead of allopathic medical approaches (like an M.D. uses). Naturopathic doctors believe nothing can cure disease but the body itself, and that nutrition is the most important factor influencing health and disease. Nutrition therapy has top priority. Allopathic doctors -- conventional medical doctors -- believe chemical/drug therapy and cutting and removing have top priority. They treat symptoms instead of causes.

147

Dr.Airola describes disease as a health restoring activity, not a negative process but instead a positive process to restore health, to cure a sick body. "It's nature's way of getting you well! ", he says.

What are the body's own healing activities? They are: pain, fever, diarrhea, fatigue, loss of appetite, and other defensive actions aimed at restoring health by eliminating the source of the problem.

According to Dr.Airola, to create the most favorable conditions for the body's own healing forces to restore health and cure disease the first step is the removal of causes. Second, a short cleansing juice fast to help the body eliminate accumulated toxins and wastes. Next, optimum nutrition, vitamins, supplements, herbs, juices, and exercise to support the body's own healing forces. Every case has specific individual adjustments.

Total relaxation and peace of mind are imperative for effective nutritional and biological therapies. Therefore, understanding and confidence in the therapies used can eliminate anxiety and hasten healing. Other factors which interfere with healing are toxic environments and inadequate digestion and assimilation.

As a nutritionist, Dr.Airola believed every effective nutritional therapeutic program should include multiple vitamin and mineral supplements (taken with food), with possible additional vitamins A, C, E, brewer's yeast, lecithin, and kelp. And, of course, raw fruits, vegetables, and juices. When health is restored, be sure to add nuts and seeds.

Dr.Airola was a forerunner in the belief that what you eat has everything to do with your health, that nutrients are what the body has to build with to maintain and restore health. And that nutritional therapy is corrective and supportive, and should be given top priority in this disease-ridden world.

*****

"Many illnesses and diseases are brought upon ourselves through carelessness, or insufficient attention to our way of life." Dr.Jan De Vries said this in his book *Cancer and Leukemia* -- an exceptional book on alternative healing approaches for cancer and leukemia. He has cured many so afflicted and helped eliminate suffering in many more with non-aggressive natural procedures.

If a person follows a conventional approach to cancer -- removal by cutting it out, or killing of both the good and bad cells -- often the cancer will spread. A remission, a removal, a restriction of growths -- all may be followed ultimately by a reappearance. And perhaps death after much suffering.

The role of the alternative health practitioner, like Dr.De Vries, is to activate the healing mechanism everyone has and return the body to normal (stasis). Often, that which is diagnosed as incurable can be controlled instead.

According to Dr.De Vries, external cancer can be relieved or eliminated by applying castor oil repeatedly. And fibroids can be eliminated with Petaforce and high potency vitamin C. Swelling, tumors, and cancer can be eliminated with Iscador (a combination of mistletoe and viscum albums) and Petasan. A cell renewer that can overcome cancer is Petasites Officinalis, with butterbur as the main ingredient. These European remedies, used by Dr.Jan De Vries and developed by Dr.Vogel, are difficult, or impossible, to find in the United States. Why?

Maximizing profits when alleviating health problems should not be a priority. Eliminating suffering should be.

* * * * *

Another outstanding leader in the alternative health movement is Robert C. Atkins, M.D., author of four bestselling health books and a practitioner of complimentary medicine for about 30 years. He reports that, "Many huge medical studies have shown beyond a doubt that <u>low</u> cholesterol is a potent precursor of cancer." He says, "The drug and food industries are using the government to make healthy eating difficult and to outlaw your freedom to make any choice whatever in your medical treatment." In other words, he says, "They want you to eat a diet of processed food high in refined carbohydrates and sugar -- far more profitable than raw food. This forces you to take their drugs when you start to suffer the results: cancer, cardiovascular impairment, headaches, hypoglycemia, etc." Dr. Atkins is a world leader in solutions to some of the most difficult diseases.

For many health problems orthodox medicine is your best choice for treatment. Emergency and trauma treatments are superb, as an example. Also, to treat effectively it is often necessary to determine the location and extent of disease in the body, and only M.D.'s, by law, are allowed to do that.

But alternative approaches are often superior for arthritis, skin problems, asthma, some cancer, diabetes, some heart problems, chronic fatigue syndrome, hypertension, hypoglycemia, learning disabilities, PMS, enlarged prostate, headaches, multiple sclerosis, menopause problems, high blood pressure, some seizure disorders, high cholesterol, colitis, overweight, and allergies.

Dr. Atkins said, "Natural nutritional remedies are enabling agents. Avoid drugs when you can. They're blocking agents with side effects that often fight your body's normal healing processes. You'll discover the body is often capable of healing itself if you give it the right stuff."

*****

When primitive cultures adopt our civilized ways of life they get our incurable diseases. Max Gerson, M.D., said, "Stay close to nature and its eternal laws will protect you."

In the days before antibiotics, Dr.Gerson cured tuberculosis patients deemed incurable with his no salt vegetarian diet. In 1929 he cured 3 incurable cancer patients. For thirty more years he continued to develop his therapy and continued to save lives that other doctors could not. He died in 1959.

Dr.Gerson cured Dr.Albert Schweitzer at age 75 of diabetes. Dr. Schweitzer then continued to work in Africa past the age of 90. Dr.Gerson also cured Mrs.Schweitzer of lung tuberculosis. He cured and improved thousands more with his healing and regenerating therapies that are holistic and natural.

Logically, degenerative diseases require regeneration of health. The Gerson Therapy floods the body with nutrients using 20 pounds of organic foods a day, most of which becomes 13 glasses of fresh juice. It avoids sodium and adds supplements like potassium to increase

151

metabolism. It uses detoxification to eliminate wastes and toxins, and to help regenerate the liver. The body is able to regenerate and become healthy because the cells regenerate and become healthy, as a result of increased oxygen and metabolism, less toxicity, and generous high quality nutrition. The Gerson Therapy eliminates disease and prevents future disease. Some people recover just by a simple change or two to help their metabolism.

Dr.Gerson explains in his book, *A Cancer Therapy -- Results of 50 Cases,* that he sought to reactivate the body's own healing mechanism in all chronic degenerative diseases called incurable. He succeeded more than a thousand times, and his success story continues.

The Gerson Institute (619-472-7450) is in Bonita, California, and the Hospital is in Mexico.

* * * * *

Computer database information on the most effective and up-to-date treatments, alternative and allopathic, from more than 100 countries is at World Research Foundation, 15300 Ventura Blvd. Suite 405, Sherman Oaks, California 91403. Also, Health Information Network at 1-800-743-6996 and The Health Resource at 1-800-949-0090. CancerHelp is at (360) 437-2291. Self-help groups can be found through the American Self-Help Clearinghouse (201) 625-7101.

* * * * *

Medical persons, as a rule, are opposed to natural, or alternative, procedures that are safer than drugs or surgery. An outstanding exception to this is Julian Whitaker, M.D., the editor of *Health and Healing*, a newsletter/magazine. He is also the author of three books about reversing health problems naturally.

Heart disease is the most common killer in the U.S., with about one million deaths each year. *Reversing Heart Disease*, Dr.Whitaker's book, proves that it is also one of the easiest to cure or avoid. He reports that the level of vitamin E in your bloodstream is a more accurate gauge of heart attack risk than cholesterol level, and that the survival rate of patients with heart disease is increased 75% by taking Co-enzyme Q10, a European remedy. Chelation therapy is a major alternative to heart surgery, a natural alternative.

Dr.Whitaker reports that an amino acid called EDTA helps Alzheimer's patients regain usual abilities, proving it is not incurable. In his book *Reversing Diabetes* he proves that with lifestyle changes, involving mostly diet and exercise, diabetes can be controlled.

According to Dr.Whitaker, "Natural treatments cannot be patented, and represent a financial threat to the status quo." There is "longstanding irrational, negative bias within the medical profession against all things nutritional." As an example, tryptophan is an amino acid very effective for insomnia, but it has been banned by the FDA without justification. However, anyone can get it in milk, bananas, and yogurt.

"The code of conformity stifles the medical profession," he said. And, "They have a legal monopoly worth billions of dollars."

* * * * *

153

If you want to increase your energy, look more vibrant, lower cholesterol, and have a more flexible body in 30 days take lecithin, pectin found in fresh fruit, and sunflower seeds, garlic, and brewer's yeast, and eliminate animal fat, every day. After 30 days, you'll feel so much better you'll want to continue! This is what Carlson Wade has written in his book *Inner Cleansing.*

He says that "Fiber is your pot of gold at the end of the rainbow of youth." It protects against diverticular disease of the colon, irritable bowel syndrome, digestive distress, and deep vein thrombosis. Wade suggests an after breakfast tonic of fresh vegetable juice, 2 tablespoons bran, and a squeeze of lemon or lime juice, blended for 20 seconds. He also suggests that 7 tablespoons of non-processed, whole grain bran daily will end colitis problems, and produce regularity. To cleanse or unclog your digestive system, every morning pour two cups boiling water over four prunes. After a few minutes drink and eat both. (Warm water is beneficial in encouraging regularity.)

Wade says that high blood pressure, fuzzy thinking, depression, confusion, fatigue, memory lapses, cramps, tingling, sharp aches and pains, are a result of clogged arteries. Wheat germ oil (2 to 4 tablespoons daily) and 30 to 60 minutes daily exercise like walking will unclog them. Excess metabolic wastes in muscles cause aches and pains. You can eliminate these with simple exercises.

Lecithin and garlic dissolve cholesterol, which is often part of gallstones. One to eight tablespoons daily of lecithin dissolves formations of gallstones. Large amounts of garlic may do the same. Garlic is also good for rheumatism and a healthy heart. Lecithin, a soybean derivative, helps heart circulation and hardening of the arteries. It breaks down cholesterol and fat in the blood.

This results in increased energy, enhances immunity, and prevents gallstones. Take 4 to 8 tablespoons daily, and omit animal-derived food.

Arthritis, according to Wade, is an imbalance of calcium and phosphorous.

Take fresh unprocessed juice daily to be healthier, he says. Currant juice washes away waste products in the liver and digestive organs. Grapefruit juice improves the health of your liver. Pineapple juice is especially rich in enzymes like bromelain. It dissolves accumulations of wastes, acting as an internal cleanser. Fresh juices help anyone look younger, live longer, and detoxify their body. Kidney, prostate, and bladder problems are cured and prevented by drinking cranberry juice daily. Apple juice washes away viruses. Prune juice cleanses your digestive system. Cabbage juice helps ulcers and their complications.

* * * * *

The book *Healing Nutrients,* by Patrick Quillin, has a section devoted to treating AIDS successfully with natural methods. Why isn't this information given to all people with AIDS? Choices are important. This book is a wealth of information for anyone seeking more information that has been carefully researched concerning nutrition and healing.

Elizabeth Kubler-Ross says, in her book, *AIDS: The Ultimate Challenge,* "People who are doing alternative medicine are doing well. Maybe you can heal yourself. It seems that the quality of life is much higher with people doing alternative therapies. There needs to be a movement for alternatives."

Humanitarian motives should be more important than monetary gain. Why else are alternative treatments hidden, and natural medical breakthroughs hidden?

* * * * *

Maureen Salaman's book, *Foods That Heal*, took about twelve years to complete. She explains ways to prevent or reverse more than 100 common ailments of varying severity. As an example, vitamin E, she says, can alleviate all problems connected with menopause, instead of using female hormones which can contribute to cancer developing. Also, hyperfunctioning thyroid problems are greatly helped by vitamins E, D, and C, and essential fatty acids (EFA's). And low functioning thyroids need kelp. Acne and eczema are helped by EFA's and zinc. Take 50 mg. zinc after each meal, three times daily, for acne. Zinc is an essential mineral for tissue repair, a healthy immune system, and healthy skin. For viruses, including herpes, hepatitis, and Epstein Barr syndrome, take 30 to 100 grams of vitamin C daily (1 gram=1000 mg.). To get rid of diabetes stop eating white flour, sugar, and fatty foods. Eat bananas for diarrhea. Eat a cup of pinto or navy beans daily to eliminate the need for insulin shots in adult onset diabetes. For anemia, take B12, iron, and folic acid. For candida albicans use lactobacillus acidophilus and brewer's yeast, and vitamin A. Also, eliminate sugar. For low blood sugar eat small meals of high protein, spaced to keep the blood sugar level stable. Salaman reports that fiber like oat and wheat bran, whole grain products, fruit and vegetables, and nuts, guards against intestinal tract ailments, heart and artery problems, and degenerative diseases like cancer.

156

CHAPTER X
WHY WE GET SICK AND HOW
TO GET HEALTHY

"Allopathic" medicine is synthetic medicine. Herbs, acupuncture, natural nutrition, massage, etc. have been used for thousands of years as natural medicine. Allopathic, or synthetic, medicine has been used for decades. Therefore, allopathic medicine is really the "alternative" medicine.

The government of Argentina gives pau d'arco free to people with leukemia and cancer. Free. This gesture of simplicity, honesty, and generosity for its population is clearly opposite of the United States government and its medical establishment. The Argentine political and medical establishment must not be organized against genuine health. In contrast, the seldom nationally reported Gestapo tactics of the Federal Drug Administration against practitioners of natural health would result, in this case, in a raid, confiscation, and shut-down of the Argentinean government itself! Why ? Because they are helping people solve health problems in a natural way (herbs) and taking business (money) away from conventional allopathic doctors, pharmacists, drug and chemical companies.

In his exposé, James Carter, M.D., Ph.D., reveals a shocking look at the $10 *billion* yearly high-tech heart disease industry. The AMA admitted in its official journal that 44% of all coronary bypass surgery is performed for inappropriate reasons.

Side effects from legal drugs put an estimated 1.6 million people in the hospital every year. That's 1.6

157

million people. No one has ever been hospitalized from herbs. At least 100,000 of these 1.6 million people die. Yet many millions of people continue to believe doctors are gods and drugs (chemicals) will and can heal. Chemicals that are synthetic cannot heal. Herbs can and do heal. So why do people persist in this faithfulness to drugs (chemicals)? Billions of dollars have been spent to propagandize drugs, for one. For another, a need to believe in the establishment. Convention is comforting, following the crowd seems safe, and being responsible for your own health is work. Also, herbs are not easy to buy, and the FDA mandates the use, the purpose, of each and every herb sold cannot be revealed on the packaging.

G. Edward Griffin, in *World Without Cancer,* said the FDA grants special favors to politically influential groups. Protection from monitoring by the FDA is available for a price. Cartel-oriented companies in the food and drug industries harass or destroy their free-market competitors. There are obviously vested political and commercial interests working against health.

Those who lack greed, arrogance, and power in the field of health and healing are often confronted with harrassment, intimidation, and fear.

In 1985, a prominent cancer researcher named Robert Schimke said, in a lecture to the National Institute of Health (the NIH), that chemotherapy makes cancer *worse* because cancer cells resist chemotherapy, which mimics the process of cancer itself. Another example of how the NIH isn't, hasn't been, and wasn't helping those suffering from cancer by using, and continuing to use, chemotherapy. Who does chemotherapy benefit? The medical establishment and chemical companies, both of which have *huge* (many millions of dollars) lobbying power. Cancer is a multi-billion dollar industry.

The AMA is a huge (millions of dollars) investor in American politics. Another meaning of the golden rule is -- to discover who rules follow the gold.

Natural medicine treats the cause of the problem rather than masking symptoms as chemicals in drugs do. As examples, feverfew herbs have been used for pain by indigenous people for centuries, as has motherwort for heart problems. But the FDA has made sure the medical establishment is protected from people being aware of this, or able to buy them. The FDA and the U.S. government protects the monopoly of the medical establishment, for their ultimate financial gain and political support.

Since it is nearly impossible to buy food that hasn't been combined with chemicals the dilemma for genuine health seems impossible to solve. Chemicals that cause ill-health are everywhere. We cannot seem to escape them. While striving to make important changes an individual or family can help prevent disease from developing by maintaining proper Ph balance. To do this eat only fruit in the morning, only vegetables in the afternoon, and only vegetables and protein in the evening. The protein source is nuts, eggs, seeds, fish that is chemical-free, or cottage cheese. According to Dr. M.T. Morter, jr., *Your Health, Your Choice,* it is necessary to eat 75% fruit and vegetables and 25% protein to maintain a 75% alkaline and 25% acid balance. This balance prevents disease.

Your body is too acid without enough *fresh* vegetables and fruits. A gallbladder problem indicates a need for minerals which neutralize the excess acid. Removing the gallbladder does not get rid of that problem. The reason for the problem remains.

159

The minerals in *fresh* vegetables and fruits neutralize acid. These minerals counteract problems, like gallbladder problems, by returning alkaline levels to normal and providing organic sodium.

It is an inescapable truth that whatever we put into our body is the foundation for what develops -- health or health problems.

* * * * *

Senior citizens face problems unique to them, or simply magnified from youth or middle age. There are many natural solutions to these problems. Ginkgo biloba is a general tonic and one of the best for counteracting problems resulting from aging. Hawthorne berry, magnesium, and carnitine strengthen and heal the heart, lower blood pressure, stabilize heart rhythm. Valerian is for insomnia. Vitamin C (at least 1000 mg) gives general well-being, energy, and strengthens the immune system. Ginseng gives physical energy, mental energy, general well-being, and lowers cholesterol and high blood pressure. Saw palmetto protects or restores prostate gland function.

Deficiencies of DHEA (from the adrenal glands), seratonin, CoQ10, B12, testosterone, progesterone, estrogen, and a thyroid imbalance, lead to aging. DHEA is stimulated by vitamin C, B-complex, and Siberian ginseng.

Nature provides answers to many health problems. As an example, flavonoids are strong anti-oxidants that neutralize free-radicals, which cause aging and sickness. Flavonoids are found in vegetables, fruit, wine, and tea.

160

The best source is grapeseed extract, which is 10%-15% stronger than pycnogenols. (Pycnogenols are 20% and 50% stronger than vitamins C and E.) Grapeseed extract helps prevent or improve varicose veins, collagen availability, vision, strokes, poor circulation, skin elasticity and smoothness, edema, high blood pressure, cancer, arthritis, aging, inflammation, and cardiovascular health. Unlike pycnogenol, its competitor, grapeseed comes from an easily renewable resource -- grapes. It is the only known source of gallic esters, the strongest free-radical scavenger known. Therefore, it is superior to A, C, E, selenium and pycnogenol.

Adequate collagen guarantees stable blood vessel walls. Cholesterol poses one-tenth the danger for eventual heart attacks as do unstable blood vessel walls. The issue then is not to cut down on cholesterol but to increase vitamin C on a daily basis. Another benefit is that C boosts good cholesterol (HDL) and decreases bad cholesterol (LDL) levels. It has been estimated that during the increased intake of vitamin C during the 1970's, (because of Linus Pauling's mass influence), the deaths from heart attacks dropped by about 30%!

According to *The Wall Street Journal*, February 1994, a recent *Lancet* study concluded that magnesium reduced cardiovascular deaths by 25%. So vitamin C and magnesium are essential nutrients for treatment of heart attack and prevention of heart attack.

Optimal cardiovascular health requires magnesium, vitamins C, B-complex, E, CoQ10, L-carnitine, minerals and trace elements, all for maximum health of the cells of the heart. Unlike some drugs/pharmaceuticals for heart problems and restoration, etc., these substances are very effective and have no side effects. Deficiencies lead to arrhythmias, impaired blood pumping, shortness of breath, edema, etc. According to Dr.Brian Leibovitz, editor-in-chief of the *Journal of Optimal Nutrition,* "The cost efficacy is even more impressive when compared to mechanical procedures like heart transplantation and bypass surgery that are major contributors to the spiraling cost of health care."

It has been estimated that 50% to 75% of people with heart problems need CoQ10 supplementation. It strengthens the immune system and, like grapeseed extract, protects and strengthens the cardiovascular system, gives energy, helps hypertension, and helps prevent strokes.

Milk thistle helps gallbladder, high cholesterol, hormonal imbalances, and liver problems like jaundice. Silymarin and dandelion also help gallbladder and liver problems and edema. St. John's wort has helped varicose veins, circulation, and immune dysfunction. Healthy veins and circulation are imperative to good health and to avoid aging. Gotu kola helps varicose veins, scleroderma, and cellulite. Ginkgo biloba helps circulation, relaxes brain capillaries and prevents strokes.

Macrobiotics is a way of eating food low in fat and high in anti-oxidants, followed expressly to overcome degenerative diseases. It has worked successfully for thousands of people.

Niacin and vitamin C help prevent and remove fatty deposits in arteries. It has been shown that heart disease can be an early form of scurvy. Vitamin C also produces collagen.

There are natural ways to renew and repair aging skin. Nutrients taken internally, and/or applied externally, function as anti-oxidants and cell regenerators for the skin. They are: evening primrose oil, essential fatty acids, vitamins A, C, E, and selenium, grapeseed

162

extract, chamomile, ginseng, loe vera, and external application of NAPCA and hyaluronic acid. Comfrey has allantoin in it, which stimulates cell growth.

Antioxidants are powerful deterrents to many diseases related to aging. This includes ginkgo biloba, a natural medicine for Alzheimer's prevention and treatment. (Use 40 mg. three times daily for prevention, and 80 mg. three times daily for treatment.)

All chronic ailments related to aging seem to benefit from avoiding and eliminating toxins in food, water, and air, juice fasting, internal cleansing, immune enhancement with supplements, managing or eliminating allergies, improvement of digestion, and reduction of stress. (Alzheimer's also benefits from aluminum chelation using deferoxamine.) Due to age, stress, and toxins in our environment most of us suffer from hormonal imbalances which lead to ill health. This idea applies especially to senior citizens. With supplementation of natural, *not* chemically derived, testosterone, estrogen, progesterone, DHEA, seratonin, CoQ10, B12, and thyroid supplements, many aging problems could be prevented. As an example, progesterone cream from wild yams has been shown to reverse osteoporosis, prevent hot flashes, and normalize hormonal imbalances for women. DHEA is a prohormone, a substance from which hormones are synthesized to then regulate metabolism. Mexican wild yam and aloe that is high in polysaccharides are probably the best sources. Also, amino acids counteract symptoms of the aging brain -- like depression, anxiety, and confusion.

Prostaglandins can cure or control many states of ill health. They are produced from essential fatty acids. EFA's lower cholesterol, blood pressure, and reduce the risks of heart attacks and strokes. However, linoleic acid -- the most important EFA -- is useless unless it is converted to gamma linolenic acid, which is converted to prostaglandins. Evening primrose oil is the only substance, except for human milk, which has GLA and no blocking agents to block conversion to prostaglandins. The body can produce prostaglandins most efficiently with evening primrose oil.

Lack of prostaglandins causes aging and many health problems. Evening primrose oil therapy of 2 to 4 grams per day, or 4 to 8 capsules, has resulted in significant improvements in heart disease, diabetes, arthritis, eczema, multiple sclerosis, high blood pressure, high cholesterol, alcoholism, hyperactivity, PMS, cystic mastitis, skin problems, edema, schizophrenia, cancer, and overweight. People who are overweight lose 1 to 2 pounds a week until reaching their best and natural weight, at which point the weight loss stops and stabilizes.

A multitude of health problems result from a deficiency of prostaglandins. Although cold-pressed sunflower, safflower, corn, or flaxseed oils have linoleic acid about one out of every 250 persons cannot convert this to GLA because of blocking agents. Anyway, it is nearly impossible to find those oils cold-pressed, except for flaxseed oil at health food stores. Borage and flaxseed oils have the highest EFA's. So evening primrose oil, flaxseed oil and borage oil have the potential to restore balance for everyone.

Cancer, according to Dr.Richard Passwater (biochemist), may be a common physical occurrence that is controlled by three defenses. These are: 1) the liver, which detoxifies cancer causing chemicals 2) the cell membrane, which protects against invasion by cancer causing chemicals and 3) the immune system.

164

Primrose oil provides the immune system with the raw materials for prostaglandins, thereby providing nutrients it needs. Besides that, Dr. Passwater reported that prostaglandins reduced cell division in malignant tissue and restored cell normality. Amazing.

It is obvious that if you fix one problem through natural means one or more other problems are likely to be also fixed. As an example, if you take bromelain for better digestion, or grapeseed extract, or calcium-magnesium-zinc, or B-complex, or garlic, for *any* problems, then back pain will also be reduced or eliminated. It makes sense that problems with health are not isolated, but are interrelated. The mechanism of the body is interdependent, one part upon the other.

*****

A recent report by the Health Research Group of the consumer organization Public Citizen listed these statistics on drugs labeled safe and effective by the FDA:

1) Each year 61,000 Americans develop drug-induced Parkinson's disease.
2) 163,000 Americans develop drug-induced memory loss or impaired thinking.
3) More than 243,000 people over age 55 are hospitalized each year because of adverse drug reactions.
4) More than two million Americans are addicted to tranquilizers or sleeping pills.

165

According to the Centers for Poison Control, allopathic medicines kill an average of 90,000 to 100,000 patients a year. Herbs, according to the CPC, have never harmed anyone.

The word "doctor" comes from the Latin word *"docere"* which means "to teach." Do your doctors "teach" you? I doubt it.

Former Iowa Representative Berkley Bedell said, "There is a growing army of angry people who are demanding a greater say in their health care." Of course, many people want doctors to tell them what to do so they don't have to make any decisions, or be responsible for anything. A kind of parent/child relationship. However, indifference, condescension, or hostility are usually the reaction doctors have when patients suggest alternatives. This is probably due to their parental or superior persona, their self-image.

Since each of us does not respond the same way to identical treatments, we need alternatives. (As an example, our nutritional requirements may vary as much as 700%.) Alternatives are always more safe than conventional approaches. Hydrochloric acid supplementation is an example. It helps anemia, allergies, mental disturbances, arthritis, and constipation because of increased digestion of nutrients and elimination of toxins. For diabetes HCL restores normal acidity so natural secretion of insulin can be maintained, since insulin is only active in an acid medium. Epilepsy is improved with HCL because it increases glutamine and arginine availability, thereby lessening convulsions and possibly eliminating them altogether. Valerian may also help.

People with psoriasis have shown improvement after HCL and B-complex supplementation. HCL deficiency can result in susceptibility to infections. Lactobacillus acidophilus has significant anti-bacterial action and it also protects against re-infection, unlike antibiotics. It is especially effective for vaginal related infections. Diminished HCL impairs digestion, so there is increased potential of food allergy reactions.

People with asthma probably have food allergies. In 1931 a study published in the *Quarterly Journal. of Medicine* concluded that 80% of 200 asthmatic children had subnormal levels of HCL. Why hasn't HCL supplementation been routinely prescribed by doctors *since 1931* for asthmatic children and adults? Probably because it really works and it is inexpensive. You don't get a prescription, you go to the health food store. Going to a health food store, or buying supplements through the mail, does not make pharmaceutical companies wealthier. And does not make you dependent on the authority of a doctor. This dependency on, and unquestioned authority of, doctors is what contributes to their arrogance, unresponsiveness to alternatives, and monetary wealth.

Gallbladder problems may be related to allergies, eggs being a very likely culprit. HCL deficiencies are very likely, also. Vegetarians have about half the incidence of gallstones as people who eat meat and eggs. An excess of soft drinks and sweets also seems to cause gallstone formation.

Vitamin E will completely eliminate restless legs syndrome. Vitamin E and EFA's can play a critical role in helping auto-immune disorders like multiple sclerosis, muscular dystrophy, rheumatoid arthritis, scleroderma, and Raynaud's syndrome. Selenium has helped people with muscular dystrophy.

A B6 deficiency is often found in infertile women and in multiple sclerosis patients. Carbon monoxide air pollution increases the need for B6. Therefore, it seems likely that cities with high carbon monoxide levels in the air would have more residents with MS and infertile women.

The *American Journal of Forensic Medicine. and Pathology,* 1983, reported: "When silver amalgam fillings are exposed to gingival action and oxidation the inorganic mercury in the fillings (especially class V fillings and root canals) may be converted to an organic form which may act as a neurotoxin." The report was "Etiology and Prevention of Multiple Sclerosis." The implications are obvious.

Colloidal silver is a natural antibiotic and disease fighter, disabling bacteria, fungus, and virus by suffocating them. The *Provo Herald,* February 2, 1992, reported colloidal silver was a cure for AIDS. Besides destroying disease organisms, it causes major growth stimulation of injured tissue, even changing cancer cells back to normal cells. Dr. Bjorn Nordstrom, Sweden, has been using colloidal silver for curing cancer for many years. It has vastly improved cases of mental retardation and Down's syndrome. It has stopped or reversed cases of AIDS and HIV.

One can only imagine why the benefits of colloidal silver have been suppressed since the early 1900's. It is a pure mineral element, not a drug. The EPA reports it has no toxicity and is harmless in any concentration. How many people have needlessly died or suffered, and continue to suffer and die, because of not being informed?

There is a growing loss of faith in a purely scientific approach to medicine. And in science telling us what is best to eat. As an example, for years margarine was touted as safe (low in cholesterol), and good to eat; butter, we were told, was dangerous (heart attacks, clogged arteries, etc.). The truth is that margarine is a poisonous trans-fatty acid that doubles the risk of heart attack. We have been told, for years, to use those polyunsaturated, hydrogenated oils that have proliferated on the grocery store shelves because they are much healthier than lard, etc. The truth is they are of no value to our health, and, in fact, are dangerous. They block production of EFA's and prostaglandins which are essential to health and well-being.

Trans-fats are caused by heat, light, air, and time, so use only cold-pressed oil. Olive oil is the only grocery store oil that is cold-pressed. If it doesn't say "virgin," "extra virgin," or "cold-pressed" it, too, has been heat processed up to 500°, and stored for long periods of time in light penetrating containers. Olive oil helps bile function and lowers cholesterol, besides being "safe". The saturated fat in butter and coconut oil is anti-viral, and is helpful for digesting fat. Grapeseed oil dates back to the Old Testament. European people have been using it for centuries. It contains 76% linoleic acid, is lowest in saturated fat, high in EFA's, and can be heated for cooking purposes without destroying the EFA's. Olive oil can also be heated but has few EFA's. Flaxseed oil is another oil with high EFA's, but it cannot be heated.

In 1994 a massive effort was made by the medical and pharmaceutical associations to make natural medicine (supplements) available only through prescription. This ever-more-greedy attempt to regulate more power and profits to doctors and pharmaceutical companies was defeated after many months, after many battles. It was a fight for health freedom. Natural supplements are so safe that no deaths, or serious health problems, or poisonings associated with any were reported during the same period that Prozac documented 28,000 serious side effects, 1,600 attempted suicides, and 1,300 successful suicides.

In an article in the *London Sunday Times*, April 3, 1994, Professor Hiram Caton of Australia said the AIDS epidemic was "a mirage, manufactured by scientists for big money, prestige, and politics. Eventually the hype will exhaust its credibility." Dr.Alfred Hassig of Switzerland said, "Multiple stresses on the immune system provoke reactions resulting in AIDS." He believed dietary measures could reverse the process and that death from AIDS is not inevitable. Dr.Henk Loman of Amsterdam believes impairment of the immune system may ultimately lead to AIDS because many people with AIDS do not have HIV, and many with HIV do not have AIDS. Philip Johnson, Professor of Law at the University of California at Berkeley, said the scientific establishment is distorting the facts to maximize its funding, by "doctoring" statistics and misrepresenting the situation.

Deadly Deception by Robert Willner, M.D., states emphatically that AIDS is caused by AZT, a pharmaceutical that slowly "murders" the person taking it. This includes, of course, helpless and innocent babies and children that have been diagnosed with HIV, a relatively harmless virus. AZT destroys the immune system, as does excess usage of any chemical/drug. People will and do recover from HIV but they will die, he says, from taking AZT (which is much stronger than anything used for cancer). The FDA, of course, must know this.

What accounts for this fraud, this conspiracy? An intricate web of deceit based on desire for power, greed, and money. A conspiracy of silence. Gullibility and vulnerability. And self-centered fear. When Margaret Heckler, head of Health and Human Services, said HIV was the cause of AIDS anyone looking for funding or credibility had to go along. A clear case of freedom of expression being suppressed by bureaucracy. As usual, to keep your job you must not make waves. The perpetrator of the AIDS myth is Dr. Robert Gallo, previously convicted of fraud, and seeking fame, power, and money, according to Dr. Willner.

Immune deficiency causes at least 25 diseases, all of which are now said to be AIDS. This is obviously manipulation of the public mentality which cannot be as informed as those in the medical community, with whom they -- the public -- entrust their lives and well-being.

Malnutrition, toxins that cause environmental and biological pollution of land, water, food and air, radiation, chemotherapy, excessive stress, and many types of drugs (chemicals) that are illegal and legal (prescription) cause immune deficiency that leads to illness. This explanation has been found in the *Merck's Manual* for many years. People need to be informed because education creates need, desire, and demand. Then things will change.

There is no question that natural agents can heal and chemicals destroy, therefore, avoidance of all those factors and use of natural healing agents can avoid or heal immune deficiencies.

The free-radical and immune system approach to eliminating cancer is to 1) take key nutrients daily 2) use an immune enhancer supplement like DHEA, shark cartilage, una de gato, echinacea, etc. The *Merck's Manual*, standard medical reference guide, states that impaired cellular immunity is involved in the growth and spread of cancer, and that the health of the immune system is essential in treating cancer and for sustained recovery. Yet, the standard treatment approaches of chemotherapy and radiation have a devastatingly destructive effect on the immune system.

171

Instead we must activate and repair the immune system. This is essential for all dysfunctional immune-system related diseases, and is simply common sense. It, however, does not make the medical and chemical establishment rich.

Phycotene, an extract from sea algae, stimulates tumor necrosis factor by 500%. DHEA, a product of adrenal hormones once available at health food stores, but removed by the FDA and now sold by the millions by prescription only, (does this surprise you?), has been used very successfully for AIDS. It enhances the immune system in general, besides helping chronic fatigue and aging. (Even a happy face and peace of mind activate the immune system!) Pau d'arco is a great immune enhancer, besides being anti-fungal, anti-yeast, and correcting many health imbalances. Una de gato is another great immune enhancer, that also helps insomnia and many other chronic health problems. Siberian ginseng and fo-ti help the adrenal glands, besides the blood and liver.

The body is a self-healing organism that benefits from support to its normal processes that have been compromised. As an example, gotu kola increases circulation and utilization of oxygen, una de gato can stop or reverse pathology, and bladderwrack supports and normalizes the thyroid. Also, the body produces estrogen from natural progesterone (not synthetic) so supplemental estrogen probably wouldn't be necessary.

Allergic reactions can be misdiagnosed as other problems. Herbs, like boswellia, stop allergies and arthritis pain with no side effects like drugs cause.

* * * * *

We are leaving the Age of Pisces and beginning the Age of Aquarius. This occurrence of astronomy and astrology should subconsciously influence people to be more concerned about their fellow man, other living creatures, and our world, with justice and equality for everyone. This sounds terrific and would certainly be an improvement.

Most governments, including the United States, are much more concerned about the economy than public health. All chemical companies are more concerned about their profits than public health. The medical establishment is more concerned about their monetary profits than public health and health of the individual.

As an example, it has been proven repeatedly that a buildup of highly carcinogenic nitrosamines causes cancer in animals and human beings. These nitrates are used to preserve hot dogs and other processed meats. Children can get leukemia if they consume too many hot dogs, studies have shown. So why aren't processed meats taken off the shelves in stores and never manufactured again? Obviously, because of the money, the profit, to be made, and political support.

Another example concerns Canada. The Canadian government revealed on national television that Monsanto, the manufacturer of bovine growth hormone to put into dairy products, attempted to bribe Health Canada with $2.5 million in 1990 if it would approve the drug.

If you would like to make a difference by promoting positive changes in our health care system and putting an end to very cruel and unnecessary animal experimentation contact Physician's Committee for Responsible Medicine, 5100 Wisconsin Ave. N.W., Suite 404, Washington, D.C. 20016.

In Europe doctors are more open to alternative approaches, saving their patients much money and suffering. The *New York Times* reported a Polish girl was given carnitine, a naturally occurring substance that metabolizes fatty acids, instead of a needed heart transplant. Her brother had had a heart transplant and died. She, however, regained normal health. Think for a moment about the magnitude of this and apply it to yourself and others you love and know. Supplementation offers great hope.

Mitral valve prolapse is a defect in the mitral valve of the heart which causes blood vessels in the head to expand resulting in headaches. About 80% of MVP people have magnesium deficiencies. Since magnesium maintains the tone of blood vessels, taking it would help the headaches. MVP indicates a magnesium, EFA, and B6 deficiency, and possibly the presence of a candida overgrowth. It is supposedly a routine procedure, more or less, to operate for this problem. I have MVP and have used B6, pau d'arco, and magnesium to great advantage. My advice based on personal experience is to try supplements before the knife. A well-known reporter, in his late 40's, died in 1995 because of a dislodged candida mass subsequently lodging in his newly installed heart valve.

Many chronic health problems/diseases are metabolic in origin. So are many common health problems. This includes mental illness and behavior problems. Therefore, problems with elimination, assimilation, absorption, circulation, digestion, nutrition, result in allergies and imbalances which lead to chronic or common health problems. As an example, lengthwise ridges on fingernails, or hair like wire, indicate mineral deficiencies. Or, zinc supplements can lessen hair loss.

Or, swelling can be caused by allergies, inadequate blood flow, or chemical sensitivities/allergies. Mental illness or behavior problems can be caused by allergies, chemical sensitivities, hypoglycemia, or candida. Nutrition and supplements can often improve these problems safely and quickly.

Energy and vitality are improved with better digestion. Better digestion results from taking betaine hydrochloric acid, lactobacillus acidophilus, and enzymes. For those suffering from petrochemical overload/allergies selenium supplements should help. Essential fatty acids like linseed oil, flaxseed oil, and evening primrose oil will get rid of rashes and eczema. *Any* health problem will improve with increased intake of oxygen. To improve memory and dream recall, and gallbladder problems, take 50 mg. to 400 mg. of B6. Deep breathing, exercise, bioflavonoids, and B6 help edema. Celtic sea salt is an unparalleled source for difficult to get trace minerals. Vitamin E increases oxygenation, delays cell aging, and causes vascular improvement. It's good for blood clots, fat metabolism, and weight loss. Calcium-magnesium helps muscle spasms. Probably every adult has a need for extra C, E, B-complex, calcium, magnesium, zinc, and D. To protect against heart attack take fish oil, magnesium, garlic, niacin, vitamin C, taurine, and carnitine. Bromelain helps upper respiratory infections, eliminates microscopic parasites and inflammation.

Comfrey has allantoin in it which enhances cell growth. Garlic and black walnut eliminate worms and parasites. Kelp helps edema, contains 28% chelated minerals, and reduces toxic radiation buildup. To help autism eliminate wheat, milk, sugar, and take B-complex with extra B6. Use chlorophyll for natural chelation.

175

Stress causes an abnormal Ph balance. So does the inevitable buildup of toxins. The result is an inability to absorb nutrients because there is too much acid and not enough alkalinity. Changing diet may relieve stress-related health problems. Massage, heat and water (hydrotherapy), exercise, and sweating (sauna), remove toxins by stimulating the lymph glands and muscles to release them. Juice fasting and intestinal cleansing are imperative. Eliminating or avoiding, or at least lessening, chemicals/toxins from our bodies is essential to restoring health and avoiding future problems. This includes removal of amalgam (52% mercury) dental fillings. And requesting alternative filling material in the future. As a matter of fact, when faced with an unsolvable health problem, this might be the missing piece of the puzzle, the solution. A man who was dying of cancer subsequently lost his teeth (with their fillings) and his cancer condition, within six months, disappeared.

It is important to treat the reasons for the problems, not just the symptoms. Physiological or chemical imbalances cause mental and behavior problems, and physical health problems. Correct the imbalances to correct the problems. The Biological Immunity Analysis is a simple evaluation of urine and saliva to determine where and what problems are, or will be, in the body. Contact the Biological Immunity Research Institute about this test to determine body chemistry balance at 1-800-321-6917.

Female hormone imbalances are best corrected with naturally occurring hormones in herbs and plants. Alfalfa has phytoestrogens. Black cohosh, dong quai, ginseng, wild yam, and sarsparilla provide natural balance. Excess estrogen that is not natural causes an imbalance that can result in many problems. The body struggles to gain

176

balance. Excess artificial estrogen reduces oxygen levels in all cells, but progesterone that is natural restores proper oxygen levels. Stress and anger cause a buildup of acid which leads to arthritis and joint pain. Yucca may be very helpful. Most importantly, though, reduce or eliminate the source of the stress or anger (which may be a hormone imbalance!).

Probably as many as 100 million people in the United States have overgrowth of candida albicans (yeast). Candida bacteria occurs naturally in everyone, but as a result of anti-biotics ("against life"), stress, diet, etc. it can easily proliferate out of control. To treat it medical doctors first have to be willing to acknowledge it. They can prescribe Nystatin, which was discovered by two sisters (microbiologists) in some dirt in New York state - thus the name Nystatin, or Nizarol, both of which are anti-fungal medications. They may need to be taken for up to two years.

Natural solutions include large doses of C, increased gradually until diarrhea begins and then decreased to tolerance level. All immune deficient disorders -- cancer, allergies, AIDS, HIV, etc. -- may need natural supplements in large doses. For candida take EFA's (flaxseed oil or evening primrose oil) at least one tablespoon daily. Also, eat no yeast, no sugar, no fat, and use vitamin-mineral supplements, pau d'arco, or una de gato, garlic (a stronger anti-fungal than Nystatin!), and HCL, lactobacillus acidophilus, and enzymes. Avoid cigarettes, smoke, and chemicals. Exercise daily, like walking or climbing stairs for twenty minutes. Last, but definitely not least, do colon-intestinal cleanses because the highest percentage/concentration of candida live in that area (about 30%).

For some people lactobacillus acidophilus will not survive in stomach acids long enough to get through the stomach, and then establish themselves in the intestine. (Normal stomach acids will burn your skin.) One solution is to use enteric coated capsules, instead of gelatin coated. If you are taking HCL, because of inadequate stomach acid, and to establish the fundamentals of digestion and absorption, take lactobacillus acidophilus at least a half an hour before taking the HCL.

A book called *The Yeast Connection,* by William Crook, has a long test for his readers to determine the likelihood of having a candida overgrowth problem.

It is important to remember this: Chemically produced imitations of naturally occurring products are potentially dangerous. Don't fool with Mother Nature! An example of the potential danger from chemically produced imitations of a natural product is L-tryptophan produced by a petrochemical company in Japan. Their so-called "natural" product never was. It was a chemical sopy. The chemical product was not processed properly, apparently, and caused 36 deaths in the late 1980's. Also, thousands of people suffered debilitating health problems. L-tryptophan is a naturally occurring amino acid in milk. Best to rely on whole foods, herbs, 100% natural supplements, or food supplements like the following group of "super-foods ":

Algae is the most basic and primitive source of pure protein, chlorophyll, chelated minerals, amino acids, and glycogen. It has worked wonders for thousands of people, balancing the system in a most effective way, resulting in energy and well-being.

Other "super foods" that are pure, unprocessed, requiring little for digestion and assimilation, and are very high in nutrients, are spirulina, chlorella, barley grass juice, wheat grass juice, kelp, dulse, de-oiled soya lecithin, apple pectin fiber, and royal jelly. All immune deficiencies are greatly helped with green foods. Chlorella, spirulina (algae), and barley grass cleanse, renew, detoxify, and energize your body.

Dr. Hagiwara, M.D., researched and developed over thirty years the "perfect natural food." This barley grass supplement is distributed and made by Green Foods Corporation in California. Barley juice has the most active ingredients of all green plants, and is thought by Dr. Hagiwara to be the very best food supplement for health.

Natural treatments to restore health, not treat the symptoms, may take months to be completed. Treatment for anemia with iron supplements, as an example, takes six to seven months to restore tissue to normal iron levels. Children with iron deficiencies may crave dirt and paint. To eliminate toxins that have accumulated for years, to facilitate the use of natural treatments, it is necessary to purify the blood, and cleanse the colon and liver. Renée Ponder, master herbalist, spent many years developing a fresh organic herb cleansing program (1-800-684-3722).

Products that are especially noteworthy for restoring balance and alleviating health problems are as follows: 1) Pau d'arco (immune enhancer and restorer of balance) 2) Una de gato (alleviation of problems and stabilization) 3) Homozon, Arise & Shine, psyllium (intestinal and colon cleanser, oxygenation) 4) Siberian ginseng (blood sugar and health balance) 5) Essiac tea, Flor•essence (diseases and immune dysfunction) 6) Lactobacillus acidophilus, enzymes (bromelain, etc.), hydrochloric acid (digestion and assimilation, elimination, allergies) 7) Aloe vera that is high in mucopolysaccharides (balance and restoration) 8) "Super-foods" like barley grass and chlorella (balance) 9) Colloidal silver (balance, restoration, infections) 10) Willard Water (balance) 11) Vitamin C, at least 500 mg. (general health and allergies) 12) Ginseng (multi-purpose) 13) Vitamin E, 400-800 IU's (heart, complexion) 14) Garlic (cholesterol, multi-purpose) 15) Brewer's yeast (multi-purpose) 16) Mexican yams, sarsaparilla, dong quai (hormone balance) 17) Kelp (thyroid balance).

Metabolic functions must be working normally. If they are not, the first step towards successful health restoration must be to restore those functions. If they are not restored no amount of money, time, and/or effort will yield more than temporary results. The most expensive health supplement won't work when the body is unable to assimilate, digest, absorb, circulate, and then eliminate, normally and adequately.

* * * * *

After having read at least 300 books and other published sources of information regarding health issues over the last three years, it has become clear that most illnesses (chronic and temporary) would benefit greatly from support and restoration of the immune system, the liver, blood, digestion, elimination, and hormone balance. Better yet, eliminate the causes to prevent most sickness.

The interconnectedness of all life forms must be understood and appreciated. We need to have a more loving, harmonious future. The body has a natural ability to heal itself. All of us, as human beings, have the power to heal ourselves, each other, and our planet.

Everybody wants happiness for themselves and those they love. Happiness is found in giving, loving, acceptance, helping others, removing stress, and simplifying our lives. It is found in yourself, not through someone or something else. But without health happiness is not possible.

*****

CHAPTER XI
LIFE IS A MATTER OF WHAT YOU BRING TO IT AND WHAT IS ALREADY THERE

The health care system in the United States is seriously flawed. But people don't know where to turn for answers and alternatives. People today show more responsibility for maintaining their health. If they demand prevention and alternatives they'll get them.

Many authorities have expressed belief that health care costs can be slashed by preventive services, preventive education, and disease preventive diets. Our health care system, costing nearly a trillion dollars yearly, has not given us healthier lives.

By the year 2000, the cost of health care will probably double. Health care is an issue most Americans want addressed. The League of Women Voters, for instance, has built grassroots support for basic health care reform, while providing community education on existing alternatives. Also, they have pushed for legislation to protect water, air, and food production, and natural resources. Joining a powerful organization like this can help you get, as the League of Women voters says, "Maximum result for your effort. Take back the system with effective activism."

European countries support alternative health care and health practitioners. It is interesting to note that when conventional doctors go on strike in other countries mortality rates drop by as much as 50%.

Thomas Edison said, "The doctor of the future will give no medicine, but will interest his patients in the care of the human frame, in diet, and in the cause and prevention of disease."

Holistic health practitioners help prevent suffering and help heal existing problems. The methods and approaches are natural, not drug-oriented. They build and restore health by dissolving and eliminating toxicity, degenerative cells, and causes of diseases by fasting, correct diet, and internal cleansing which ensures proper cell and bodily waste elimination, and improvement and maintenance of health. Effective natural treatments for ailments and preventive care are incorporated.

In a letter to me Congressman Baker of Louisiana said, "An affordable health care reform option is important. It is important that we expand consumer choice and that we emphasize preventive care."

*****

Prevention is better than cure. Who can dispute this? However, as an acquaintance of mine related, "People are more interested in dealing with health problems after they occur, and not preventing them." The American Cancer Society recently reported that more than one million people a year are diagnosed with cancer, involving 3 out of 4 families. *In the United States, someone dies from cancer every minute.* MANY BILLIONS OF DOLLARS in research have not prevented cancer becoming like a communicable out-of-control disease. Obviously, something is drastically wrong about our society, which causes cancer, and about our medical establishment, which cannot prevent or cure cancer.

We do not have to be victims. We are not helpless. We CAN avoid many illnesses and diseases. We CAN

183

eliminate, or lessen the severity of, many illnesses and diseases. There ARE alternative approaches to health which work.

The *New England Journal of Medicine* reported calcium supplements *reverse* the spread of colon cancer cells, returning them to normal within 2 to 3 months. Every person with colon cancer should be told this, routinely, by his/her doctor.

Nearly half a million Americans a year are candidates for heart transplant surgery because of cardiomyopathy, or heart failure. A wonderful alternative about 80% of the time is Co-enzyme Q10, a nutrient available at health food stores and vitamin suppliers. It's a natural substance so it can't be patented. This means no money for research, no massive profit potential, no promotion from big drug companies and doctors, and no acknowledgement from the medical establishment that would stand to lose billions of dollars. The suffering, agony, and pain are obviously of no consequence. It costs about $40 a month for Co-enzyme Q10 compared to about $150,000 for each heart transplant.

A cause of chronic fatigue syndrome is B-complex deficiency. Drug treatment makes it worse. People with chronic fatigue can get Social Security benefits. Imagine -- for easily fixed nutritional deficiencies! The medical establishment feeds government programs and government programs feed the medical establishment.

The health care industry doesn't want you to know about treatments that won't bring them money. And doctors don't want to be labeled as outsiders by their peers or by the American Medical Association. How many doctors would rather see a patient suffer or die than be cured by alternative therapies?

184

A *New England Journal of Medicine* study in 1993 reported that, "One in three Americans now use alternative therapies."

"Modern technology has addressed itself well to the traumatic and acute needs of people, but it has done little . . . to promote wellness and holistic health." -- Dr. Chester Yozwick.

Alternative therapies follow what Hippocrates, the father of medicine, said -- "Above all do not damage." Modern medical technologies follow the cut, radiate (X-ray), and chemical (drug) approach. Damage is inevitable. Anyone who is sick or in pain doesn't want, or need, treatments that harm them. Anyone who is healthy doesn't want treatments that harm them. Yet, Western medicine consistently does exactly that. Oriental medicine, Indian medicine (Western and Eastern), holistic medicine, and Naturopathy use only therapies that enhance healing, that enhance health. We need to support the human body to maintain, and regain, balance, not cut, destroy, and increase the imbalance.

Anything in the human system that goes out of harmony will cause problems. Emotions, excess stress, and physical trauma greatly influence the endocrine glands, affecting the hormonal balance, and ultimately your immune system. The balance of health obviously can be upset by modern medical techniques and technologies.

To avoid problems developing we need to eliminate excessive stress -- mental, nutritional, environmental, physical.

Americans are seeking alternatives to traditional medicine. In 1990, Americans spent $13.7 billion on alternative medicines and treatments, $10 billion not covered by insurance. American people are obviously interested in natural ways to improve their health.

There are multiple approaches to health and sickness. Maximizing profits should not be a priority -- eliminating suffering should be.

Joseph Califano, former Secretary of HEW, said in his book *Radical Surgery*, "Health care is above all a ministry, not an industry, and we, as well as doctors and nurses, have an obligation to minister to our own health." But in reality the medical bureaucracy and sickness <u>are</u> an industry, a very lucrative part of the economy.

Every person's physiological and mental self is the same as, yet certainly different than, someone else's. What benefits one person may not benefit the other. Be receptive, therefore, to alternatives. Everyone has inherited strengths and weaknesses unique to each individual, which respond to lifestyles, medical therapies, and environment in their own unique way.

The autonomic nervous system stimulates organs and glands to function, resulting in chemical and hormonal production. This in turn affects personality and physical characteristics. The reaction of our body's life processes to enzyme activity is our metabolism. Metabolism is the exchange of energy (heartbeat, digestion, circulation) with elements of the environment. How a person uses these elements to maintain life differs from one person to another.

Life is a matter of what you bring to it and what is already there. We are as unique on a metabolic level as we are in our fingerprints. Therefore, individual needs are different.

* * * * *

It is human nature to strive to be happy, productive, and loved. It is necessary to be physically and mentally healthy to achieve this.

We need to follow a natural way of life that leads to natural health and well-being. Not chemically induced and sustained pseudo-health, and pseudo-well-being.

When people become more unified and vocal in their opposition to massive pollution of the Earth, the air, the water by multi-billion dollar industries, more progress will be made toward stopping it and restoring the balance of Nature. This, of course, affects our mental, physical, and spiritual balance, individually and collectively.

Anyone can save thousands of dollars and untold suffering by taking charge of their own health and sharing knowledge of health methods. Holistic or natural health restoration and maintenance will result in a healthier, longer, and happier life.

Why is it necessary to "scientifically" prove things? Science is, and has been, fraught with error. We may not be able to "prove" how alternative health approaches work, so we just have to accept that they do and be grateful.

Medicine is defined in Webster's dictionary as: "The science and art dealing with the maintenance of health and the prevention, alleviation, or cure of disease." Medicine and healing need to be insight and knowledge combined with compassion for the whole self -- body, mind, and spirit (or soul).

Restoration of health is possible with the methods described in this book, as a result of better circulation, better blood quality, a better functioning metabolism, liver and digestive system, and a more effective immune system.

The causes of disease must be removed and the conditions of health established. People can be guided to superior health by helping them understand, by modified fasting, by correcting nutrition, by eliminating chemicals and excessive stress, by drinking pure water, by breathing fresh unpolluted air, with regular exercise like walking, and adequate sunshine and sleep. A natural way of life.

"To attain knowledge, add things everyday.
To attain wisdom, remove things everyday."
-- Lao Tsu

* * * * *

AFTERWORD

Whatever happens in our lives reflects the potential for mental, emotional, physical, or spiritual growth. Death is the release of spirit, of consciousness, to another level of understanding, to another plane of existence, another dimension. All present experiences are related to all past actions -- going back to the beginning of our individual creation. We are a combination of all that has come before.

If the purpose of life is to increase love and wisdom, and God is love, then the purpose of life is spiritual -- not materialistic or physical. For the most part, Man is out of harmony with his universe, with Mother Earth. Health problems are a direct result. Since science is materialistic and physical, and not spiritual, science has not and will not restore that harmony that it has disrupted. Science focuses on external observations, not the purpose of life, not balance and harmony.

Yin and Yang are action and reaction -- Balance. For every action there is a reaction -- Balance. Love creates balance, balance creates love. Change enables us to redefine ourselves and our lives. Change is the process by which we evolve on this plane of existence. Change awakens us to a new way of being. We need to establish physiological, mental, emotional, and spiritual balance to have genuine health. Most of us need to incorporate change into our lives to achieve this.

Every generation since humanity began is a modern generation because it follows an older generation. "Modern" is not synonymous with "better" or "improved".

I predict that ancient Oriental medicine will become more widely appreciated, accepted, and used, as our society becomes less enchanted with our traditional Western medicine, and more open-minded about others.

Ancient Chinese medical approaches balance the energy (qi) in the body. Blood is the source of energy. The liver is the primary regulator, the source of balance and the life force (qi), along with the spleen, the heart, the kidneys and the lungs. Disharmony between them causes most health problems and can be corrected with herbs and acupuncture, methods used successfully for about 2,500 years. Oriental methods are painless, poison-free, and productive. Western methods are often full of pain, poisons to kill that pain and bacteria, and destructive.

As an example, diabetes, in China, is not a disease but a blood sugar, pancreas, digestion imbalance which can be corrected with herbs. As another example, Western medicine removes a prolapsed uterus (extremely painful and usually causing problems to develop for years). Eastern medicine, on the other hand, strengthens the spleen and liver with herbs and acupuncture (no pain, improving health [balance] instead of destroying it), and thereby corrects the prolapse. Also, Chinese medicine has been using shark cartilage to cure cancer and heart disease for about 100 years. Here, it's still being tested for effectiveness.

As Victor Hugo said, "Will the future ever arrive?"

It seems that lasting happiness is found from helping others and forgiveness, from having a purpose to fulfill for your days and life in general, from making a choice to be happy, from giving and kindness, from appreciation for what you have. But if you're not healthy most of this is impossible. Happiness is also dependent upon good health.

* * * * *

It is my hope that people will learn something important from my book. Something to improve their life, and other lives. I thought of naming it *Therapeutic Nutrition -- The New Medicine.* But I realized I would be treading on sacred ground and a monopoly. Physicians get very upset when anybody else alludes to the possibility of "practicing medicine." (Just look at all the disclaimers on health supplement booklets, etc., as an example.) The wrath of these gods may be upon me. The AMA may sue me in revenge! The drug industry may retaliate! All because I used the "M" word -- "medicine", a word which has taken on the meaning of money and mystery and monopoly. "Medicine" is a profession, a religion, of which only supposedly God-like creatures -- doctors -- can say they know the secrets thereof. Beware the heretics and infidels who tread their sacred ground. Too many medical doctors have become self-proclaimed gods in their heavens of power, monopoly, greed, and money.

For approximately the past 100 years the medical establishment has tried to reinvent the wheel. Invasive methods (painful) and chemical methods (destructive) are not the answer. They have too often caused immense suffering instead of relieving it, costing untold trillions of dollars in the process. We have been victims, therefore, for a very long time.

Medical doctors do not heal. Only the body itself, and Nature, can heal. That inherent healing ability must be stimulated, not depressed by poisons (synthetic drugs), cutting (traumatic surgery), and burning (radiation).

Suppression of positive results from other healing disciplines by the FDA and AMA, and legal punishment

191

by the FDA and AMA of any remote possibility of "practicing medicine" with alternative modalities, will cease when people become more informed and support alternatives.

In times of ill health medical doctors offer us hope. But too often it is a false hope. Their solutions create problems. As an example, the huge number of women with hysterectomies in the U.S. is connected with the huge increase in breast cancer and heart disease. All three are multi-billion dollar industries. In and of themselves, hysterectomies, like other radical procedures, often create more problems than they solve. Do medical doctors avoid these same procedures for themselves?

We need choices, not commands or ultimatums. The whole person must be taken into account -- Body, Mind, and Spirit. This, in turn, fosters a holistic attitude towards all of life. Each one of us, after all, has responsibility for our society, our environment, our selves. Your health is your most valuable possession. Without it, nothing else really matters.

* * * * *

APPENDIX

The best sources -- prices, courtesy, quality -- for supplements and herbs, or for more information about natural holistic health, (other than sources previously mentioned), are:

Swanson's 1-800-437-4148
Biotrition   1-800-430-5023
Beres Drops Plus 1-800-294-8787
Vitamin Power 1-800-645-6567
Vitamin Shoppe 1-800-223-1216
L & H Vitamins 1-800-221-1152
Dyna-Pro 1-800-877-1413
Nature's Distributors 1-800-624-7114
Future Med 1-800-800-8849

Recommended publications that support alternative health are:

"Second Opinion", P.O. Box 467939, Atlanta, GA
  31146-9989
"What Doctor's Don't Tell You", 105 West
  Monument Street, P.O. Box 17477, Baltimore, MD
  21298-9016
"The Spotlight", 30 Independence Avenue S.E.,
  Washington, D.C. 20003-1081
"Nexus", 1680 Sixth Street, Boulder, CO 80302
"Co-op America", 2100 M Street N.W., Washington,
  D.C. 20063

Information resources for chronic health problems:

The World Research Foundation (818) 907-5483
The Health Resource 1-800-949-0090
The Health Information Network 1-800-743-6996

Alternative health centers:

International Medical Center 1-800-621-8924
Alternative Cancer Therapies (213) 663-7801
Cancer Treatment Centers of America
1-800-234-0490
American Biologics-Mexico 1-800-227-4458
Center for the Improvement of Human
Functioning (316) 682-3100

BIBLIOGRAPHY

1. *Can We Contain Health Care Costs ?*, Jennifer Baratz.

2. *Keeping Environmental Toxins At Bay*, S. Lancer, M.D.

3. " The Evolution Time Bomb " Paul Pritchard, *National Parks Magazine*, August, 1993.

4. *The 50 Healthiest Places to Live And Retire in The U.S.,* Norman Ford.

5. " The Energy Times, " vol. 3, no. 2 *Organic Food.*

6. *Say No to Cancer*, Barbara Waters.

7. *Silent Spring*, Rachel Carson.

8. T.C. Frye Publications.

9. *Healing Nutrients*, Patrick Quillin.

10. *Do Miracles Exist ?*, Jan De Vries, M.D.

11. *Viruses, Allergies, and The Immune System*, Jan De Vries, M.D.

12. *Back to Eden*, Jethro Kloss.

13. *Arthritis, Rheumatism, and Psoriasis*, Jan De Vries, M.D.

14. *Cancer and Leukemia*, Jan De Vries, M.D.

15. *The Hysterectomy Hoax*, Stanley West, M.D.

16. *Louisiana Out of Doors*, newspaper publication.

17. *The Un-medical Book*, Elizabeth Baker.

18. *The Way of Herbs*, Michael Tierra.

19. *Our Earth, Our Cure,* Raymond Dextreit.

20. *Liver Disease and Gallstones,* Alan Johnson and
    David Triger.

21. *Limits to Medicine,* Peter Illich.

22. *The Truth About Protein,* Robert Allen.

23. *The Great White Lie,* Walt Bogdanovich.

24. *How to Prevent Pesticide Pollution,* Jeffery Dearborn.

25. *Careers for Nature Lovers,* Louise Miller.

26. *AIDS: The Ultimate Challenge,* Elisabeth Kubler-Ross.

27. " The Value of REAL SEASALT " The Grain and Salt
    Society.

28. *USA Today,* newspaper, September 27, 1993.

29. *Minerals -- How Important Are they to You ?,* Anne
    Sommers.

30. "Food Should Be Your Medicine," *Health Digest* .

31. *A Gerson Therapy -- Results of 50 Cases,* Max Gerson,
    M.D.

32. *Natural Health,* magazine.

33. *Health and Healing,* newsletter. Julian Whitaker, M.D.

34. *How to Get Well,* Paavo Airola, M.D.

35. *Tomorrow's Health,* newsletter. Robert C. Atkins,
    M.D.

36. *The Whole Food Bible,* Christopher Kilham.

37. *Foods That Heal,* Maureen Salaman.

38. *Inner Cleansing,* Carlson Wade.

39. *Diet for a New America,* John Robbins.

40. *Lifelines Magazine,* Spring, 1994.

41. *A Road Less Traveled,* M. Scott Peck, M.D.

42. *Turn Back the Clock,* newsletter. Summer, 1994. Dr. Keith Johnson.

43. *No More Hysterectomies,* Vicki Hufnagel, M.D.

44. *Enzymes,* Anthony Cichoke, D.C.

45. *Acquiring Optimal Health,* Gary Price Todd, M.D.

46. *Why I Left Orthodox Medicine,* Derrick Lonsdale, M.D.

47. *Heart and Soul,* Bruno Cortis, M.D.

48. *What Doctors Don't Tell You,* a British newsletter (pub. since 1986).

49. *Radical Surgery,* Joseph Califano, M.D.

50. *The Difference Between Men and Women,* Susan Lark, M.D.

51. *Beating Alzheimer's,* Tom Warren.

52. *Nutritional Influences on Illness,* Melvyn Werbach, M.D.

53. *Deadly Deception,* Robert Willner, M.D.

54. *Vitamin B6: The Doctor's Report,* Dr. John Ellis.

55. *The Chelation Way,* Dr. Morton Walker.

56. *Options for Alternative Cancer Therapy,* Richard Walters.

57. *Coronaries, Cholesterol, and Chlorine,* Joseph Price, M.D.

58. *Fluoride: The Aging Factor,* John Yiamouyiannis, Ph.D.

59. *Reversing Heart Disease,* Julian Whitaker, M.D.

60. *Physician's Desk Reference.*

61. *A World Without Cancer,* G. Edward Griffin.

62. *Your Health, Your Choice,* M.T. Morter, jr., M.D.

63. *Federal Catalog of Domestic Assistance.*

64. *Between Heaven and Earth,* Harriet Beinfield & Efrem Korngold, O.M.D.

Index

Jensen, Dr. Bernard, 85, 87
Joint problems, 32, 94, 103,
    104, 129, 130, 136
Jung, Dr. Carl, 59

Kelp, 59, 91, 98, 102, 116, 135,
    148, 156, 175, 179, 180
Kidney stones, 37, 40, 45, 62,
    82, 88, 102, 119, 120, 125,
    155
Kuhl, Dr. Johannes, 45

Lactobacillus acidophilus,
    50, 77, 84, 93, 122, 132, 156,
    167, 175-179
Laetrile, 65, 97
Lake Superior, 31
Lecithin, 118, 119, 123, 132,
    133, 136, 139, 148, 154, 179
Lemon juice, 43, 45, 59, 74,
    75, 117, 123, 132, 133, 135,
    138, 154
Leukemia, 15, 95-98, 103,
    106-108, 116, 137, 149, 157,
    173

Liver, 3, 7, 12, 13, 40-45, 49,
    53-56, 59, 64, 66, 74, 76, 88,
    98, 103, 107, 117, 120, 129,
    140, 152, 155, 162, 172, 179,
    180, 187, 190
London Sunday Times , 170
Louisiana, 18, 19, 31, 83, 183
L-tryptophan, 178

Macrobiotic diet, 38, 39, 72,
    96, 115, 162
Magnesium, 37, 59, 73, 89,
    91, 95, 98, 102, 107, 108,
    114, 119, 128, 135, 139, 141,
    160, 161, 165, 174, 175
Manganese, 80, 94, 103, 119,
    135
Mead, Margaret, 6, 16
Meat, 14, 21, 27, 41, 44, 45,
    48, 56, 57, 60-63, 74, 76, 94,
    122, 131, 136-139, 167, 173
Medical research, 22-27, 34,
    56, 103, 111, 121, 152, 155,
    184, 194
Medical tests, 25, 37, 89, 176,
    178
Menopause, 42, 99, 100, 104,
    123, 150, 156
Mental problems, 6, 59, 60,
    70, 71, 86, 100, 101, 105,
    117, 130, 131, 146, 160, 166,
    168, 174-176, 186

Mercury, 23, 80, 119, 135, 138, 168, 176
Metabolism, 57, 80, 81, 84, 91, 105, 108, 126, 127, 144, 146, 152, 163, 175, 186, 187,
Mexican yams, 103, 134, 163, 180
Milk thistle, 123, 133, 134, 138, 162
Minerals, 7, 22, 29, 42-45, 54, 60, 64, 71, 78-81, 86, 91, 94-98, 102, 106, 108-114, 124-131, 133, 136, 140, 141, 145, 148, 156, 159-161, 168, 174-178
Mitral valve prolapse, (MVP), 174
Montmorillonite clay (Coso), 42, 74, 106, 108, 137, 141
Morris, Nat, 98
Multiple sclerosis, 23, 94, 104, 133, 150, 164, 167, 168
Muscular dystrophy, 104, 167

National Institute of Health, (NIH), 158
Natural beauty, 3, 140
Naturopathic medicine, 139, 147, 185
Nevada, 14

New England Journal of Medicine , 184, 185
Nitrosamine, 173
Nuclear, 14, 15, 32, 76, 98

Oils, cold-pressed, 55-61, 74, 75, 81, 89, 140, 143, 164, 169
Olive oil, 55, 61, 74, 75, 81, 140-143, 169
Organic farming, 16, 18, 29, 36, 55, 69
Organic food, 16, 28, 68, 69, 76, 122, 137, 151
Overweight, 7, 12, 20, 40, 42, 83, 98, 151, 164
Oxygen, 60, 63-66, 78, 80-82, 85, 87, 96, 98, 105, 106, 117, 132, 144-147, 152, 172

Pacific Yew tree, 68
Pap smears, 25
Papaya, 77, 79, 122
Parkinson's disease, 21, 65, 102, 133, 165
Passwater, Dr. Richard, 164, 165
Pau d'arco, 65, 93, 96, 97, 102, 107, 108, 132-137, 157, 172, 174, 177, 179

Pauling, Dr. Linus, 64, 85, 125, 161
Peck, Scott, M.D., 31
Peppermint oil, 77, 120
Pesticides, 5, 15-18, 28, 31-33, 36, 42, 68, 69, 111, 127, 144
Pets, 107-110
Phenols, 61
Ph balance, 125, 142, 159, 176
Physician's Committee for Responsible Medicine, 173
Physician's Desk Reference, 33
Phytochemicals, 56, 100, 176
Picasso, Pablo, 5
Pitcairn, Dr., 109-110
Plato, 11
Potassium, 86, 95, 102-104, 109, 113, 114, 118, 128, 151
PMS, 93, 114, 134, 150, 164
Prince Charles, 20
Progesterone, 10, 11, 99, 100, 123, 160, 163, 172, 177
Prostaglandins, 77, 163-165, 169
Prostate problems, 37, 103, 130, 134, 150, 155, 160
Psoriasis, 7, 53, 93, 118, 125, 137, 166
Pycnogenols, 144, 161

Quarterly Journal of Medicine, 167
Quillin, Patrick, 155

Relman, Dr. Arnold, 37
Rheumatism, 7, 42, 46, 73, 74, 81, 114, 117, 138, 154, 167
Robbins, John, 62
Root canal, 138, 168
Ross, Elizabeth - Kubler, 155

Salaman, Maureen, 98, 156
Sarsparilla, 134, 180
Saw palmetto, 37, 103, 130, 134, 160
Schopenauer, 36
Schweitzer, Dr. Albert, 7, 56, 151
Sea salt, Celtic, 98, 113, 114, 122, 132, 137, 175

The
1-800
Health Directory

First Edition

Keeping Hope Alive

Flor•Essence™ for a Brighter Future

THE TRIED AND TRUE FORMULA

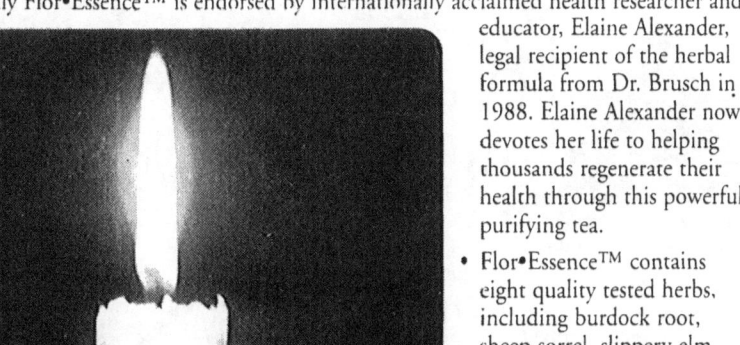

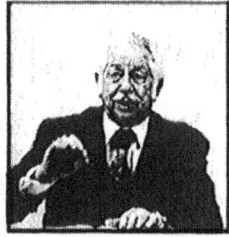
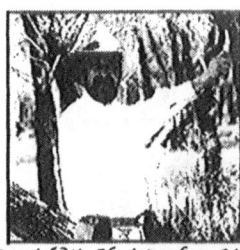

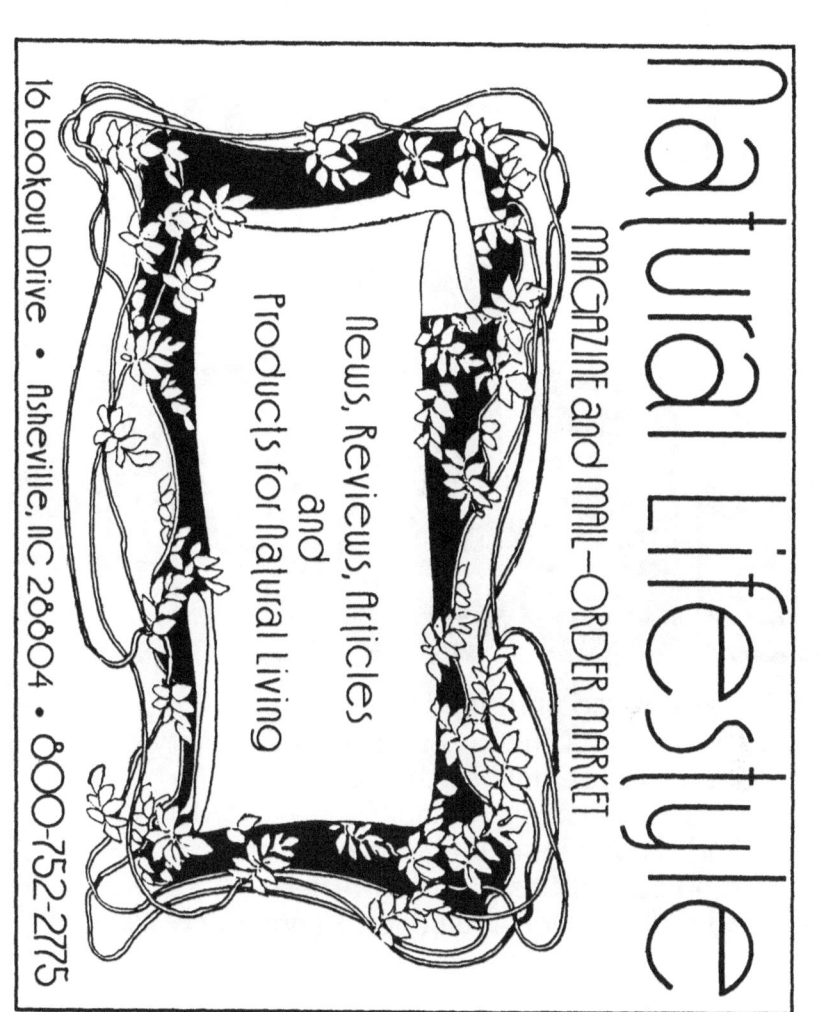

Barlean's Organic Oils

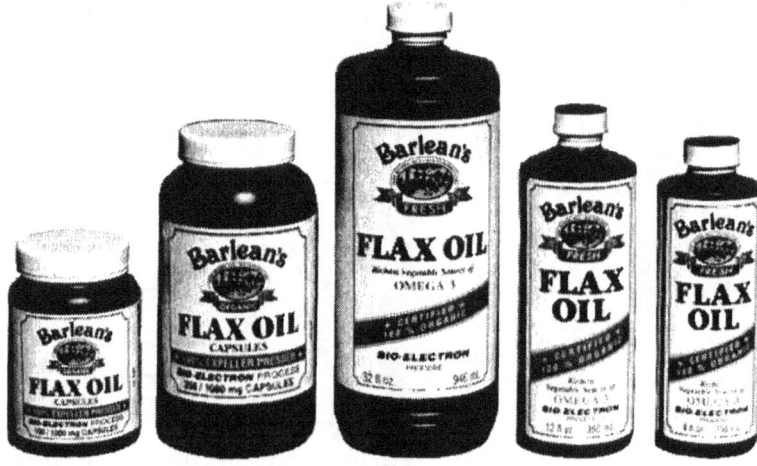

- 100% natural and unrefined
- Rich in "essential" Omega-3 and Omega-6 fatty acids, required for optimal health
- "High in Lignan" flax oil available
- The brand recommended by more health and nutrition authorities than any other
- Featured in "Healthier, Wealthier, Happier and Wise"

"There are few foods or supplements that hold the potential of Barlean's Organic Flax Oil." Jade Beutler, Author of **"Flax for Life"**.

"Barlen's Flax Oil is the brand I trust and use for my personal, family and patient use." Dr. Michael Murray, world renown natural medicine expert and author of **"Understanding Fats and Oils"**.

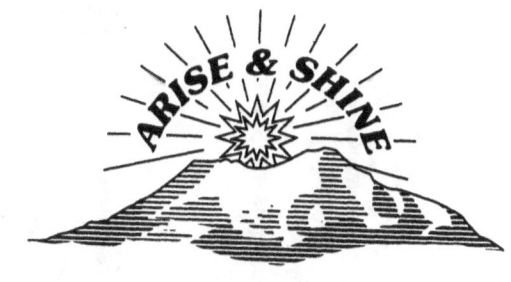

Detoxification:

The #1 Alternative For Vibrant Health

In 1986, Dr. Richard Anderson, N.D., N.M.D., was in the mountains with an herbalist friend, living off the land, eating only wild, fresh herbs. After a few days the two men began eliminating leathery material up to 4 feet in length -- they were utterly astonished! As they continued to eliminate these fecal mucoid layers, their strength and vitality surpassed anything they had ever experienced. Realizing how important this discovery was, Dr. Anderson began researching the herbs that were responsible for these incredible results. He tested and recreated, and soon CHOMPER and HERBAL NUTRITION, the foundations of the program, were born!

"I just couldn't believe what came out of me - everything from green globs to strings of black, rubbery stuff. I lost about 20 pounds of this junk! I feel so much cleaner now, and my health has dramatically improved. -- Albert C., Rhode Island

The Cleanse Thyself ™ program has helped tens of thousands of people all over the world achieve better health. Thousands of people have reported the elimination of up to 50 feet of impacted waste material after doing just one cleanse! Many who were not overweight have testified that they were totally amazed they could have had such an accumulation, and that their health and energy level could improve so remarkably.

Experience the power of "The Cleanse" yourself!

Call for a FREE catalog/info pack: **1-800-688-2444**

Arise & Shine   3225 N. Los Altos   Tucson, Arizona 85705

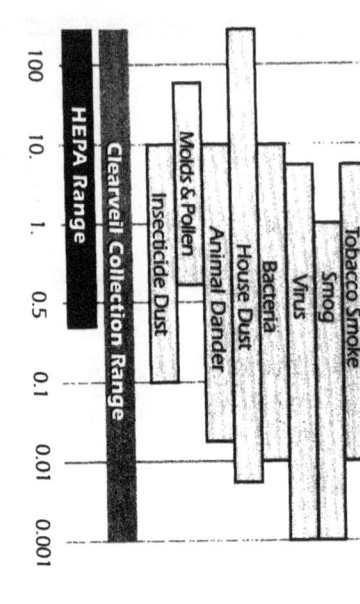

	100.	10.	1.	0.5	0.1	0.01	0.001
HEPA Range							
Clearveil Collection Range							
Molds & Pollen							
Insecticide Dust							
Animal Dander							
House Dust							
Bacteria							
Virus							
Smog							
Tobacco Smoke							

How Clearveil Works:

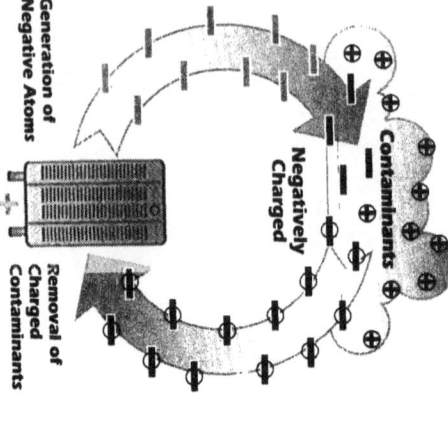

Generation of Negative Atoms

Clearveil

Contaminants

Negatively Charged

Removal of Charged Contaminants

Attention Allergy Sufferers!

Relief is here at last!

Enjoy a Cleaner, Healthier Environment With Clearveil

- Removes pollutants that can cause allergies, stress, shortened attention span, colds and flu

- Eliminates contaminants other units miss

- Small, noiseless purifier ideal for home or office

- Costs about 1¢ to operate a day

- You know it's working because the used collection sheet is covered in pollutants

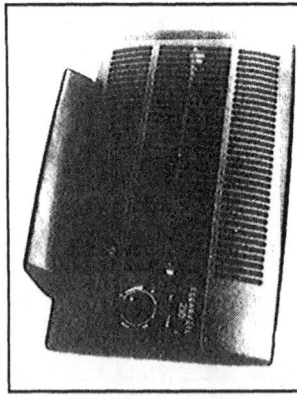

Available at:

C L E A R V E I L™

FANLESS ELECTRONIC AIR PURIFIER

4.5x3.75

Nutritional and Health Supplement Customer:

Now You've found what you've been looking for

Highest in quality and lowest in price.

Quality Standards: Before we start producing or adding any product to our line, we do the best quality research possible on all sources available.Only then we do carefully select each product in our line.

Pricing - Quality for less: Our regular retail price for one bottle is lower than all sales and specials

on the market.

The reason we can sell quality for less is quite simple We control the potentially high cost of production, distribution, and promotion.

This allows us to offer to you the cutomer, quality for less over all Discounters and Mail-order Houses.

Bulk & Specialties Crop.

152 South 9th St. Brooklyn,N.Y.11211

1-800-571-8862

Concerned about the quality of your tap water? Do you BUY bottled water?

Get the #1 rated Water Purifier

MULTI-PURE DRINKING WATER SYSTEM

* For renters or homeowners.

* *25 year warranty.* Free trial, money-back guarantee.

* Cheaper, more convenient, *safer* than bottled water.

* Removes lead, parasites, heavy metals, solvents, chlorine & carcinogenic by-products. Better than *any* other filter!

* (*ertified top rating* by NSF Intl. *and* States' Depts. of Health, Consumer Reports. Named "Best Buy" in Consumer's Digest.

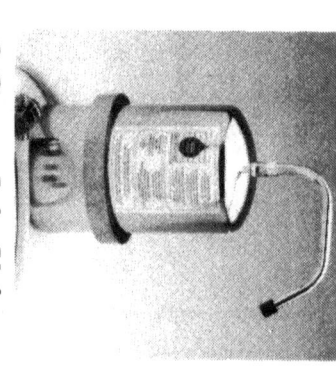

Are You Looking for Extra Income? Come Join Us!

We train and support you to successfully develop a full or part-time business through a simple, easy network marketing plan. Get your filter retail, wholesale or free. No inventory. A small investment in your livelihood today grows an abundant future. Benefit yourself, your friends, relatives, co-workers & community with unlimited purest water for life.

To Purchase or Distribute MULTI-PURE Water Filters, contact :

Pamela Crawford * WaterBearer, Inc. * PO Box 8585 * Emeryville, CA * 94662-8585

(800) 656-9399

"If you don't have this filter, YOU ARE the filter!"

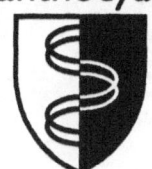

MAKE A
SICK HOUSE WELL
with the
LIVING AIR XL-15

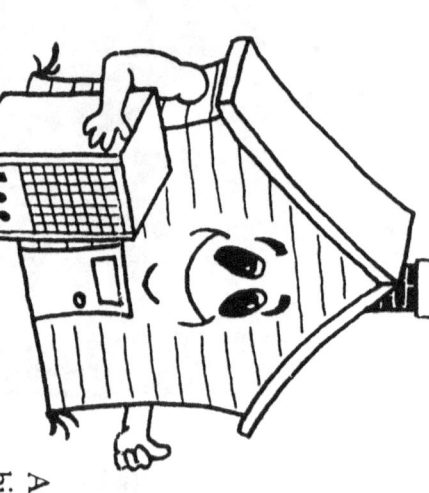

According to the EPA, indoor air pollution is our nation's biggest pollution problem. Modern homes and buildings are so energy efficient they block out nature's air cleaning agents and trap pollution inside—inside where you probably spend 90% of your time. What can you do?

Ventilation systems can be expensive, and filters provide only a partial remedy. Why not look at nature? Living Air looked to nature before designing the revolutionary XL-15, an electronic thunderstorm in a box. A thunderstorm is nature's most powerful air cleaning activity. Why not take the test? Ask for a free, no obligation demonstration of the powerful Living Air XL-15

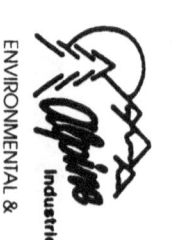

ENVIRONMENTAL &
WELLNESS PRODUCTS

IRA POFF
CONSULTANT

AIR PURIFICATION
EFFECTIVELY REDUCES
SMOKE • MOLD • BACTERIA
ODORS • GASSES • POLLEN

HEALTHIER 2000
202 OLE HICKORY TRAIL

770-888-1011

A Career in Holistic Health

Begins With Education

Bachelor's/Master's/Doctorate

If you have the desire to become a holistic health practitioner or specialize in a natural healing modality, a degree in Wellness Science is your first step. Study the foundations of physical and mental wellness through home study and acquire a thorough understanding of holistic health and healing as it relates to the integration of the body, mind and spirit.

For additional information call...

1-800-398-8484 ext 148

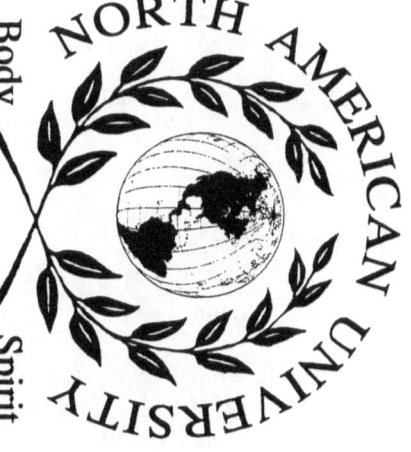

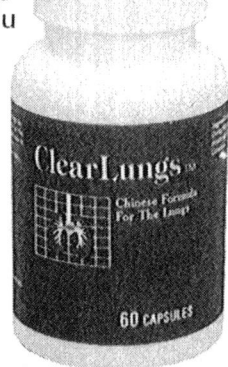

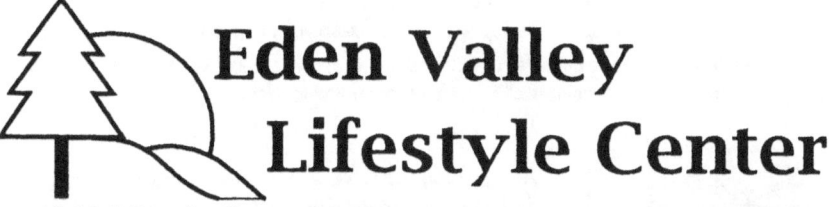

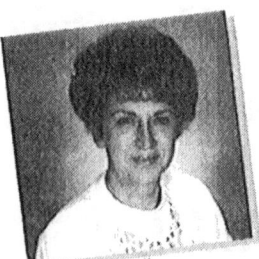
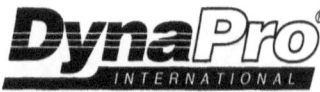

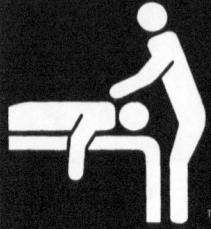
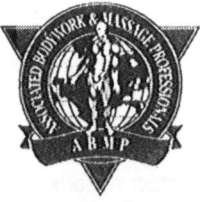

Feed Your Highest Instincts.

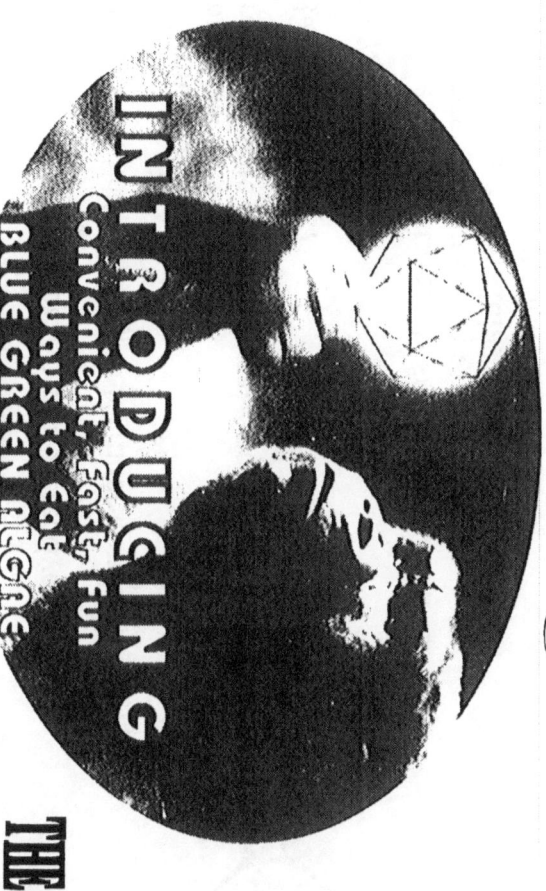

INTRODUCING
Convenient, Fast, Fun
Ways to eat
BLUE GREEN ALGAE

"The greastest value of AFA is not only its nutrient concentrations, but its effect on the nervous system... People taking AFA have reported an overall increase in mental alertness, mental stamina, short and long term memory, problem solving, creativity, dream recall, and a greater sense of wellbeing and centeredness."
Dr. Gabriel Cousens

THE ORIGINAL SUPERFOOD

Available at your local co-op and health food stores

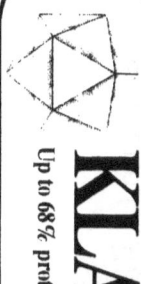

Healing Solutions
For You and Your Animal Companions

Teachings and Healing of the Miquon-Apache

Interspecies Communication

National Lost Companion Animal Detective Service

Workshops on Self Healing, Self Understanding

J.L. Running Horse
Animal Rescue Team
Search & Rescue International, Inc.
P.O. Box 907
Girdwood, AK 99587

(907) 783-3072

Telephone consultations. Distance is no obstacle.
Correspondence courses on audio cassette
Traveling seminar schedule.
Please call or write for information.

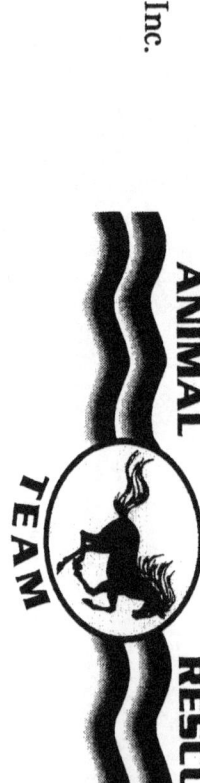

ANIMAL TEAM RESCUE

"My work is to bring human and other kingdoms
together with mutual respect and understanding."